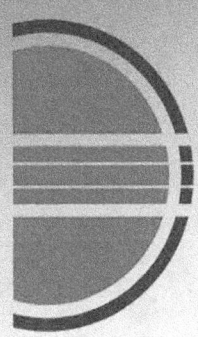

DIABETES MELLITUS
INTERAGENCY
COORDINATING
COMMITTEE

Coordinating the Federal Investment in Diabetes Programs To Improve the Health of Americans

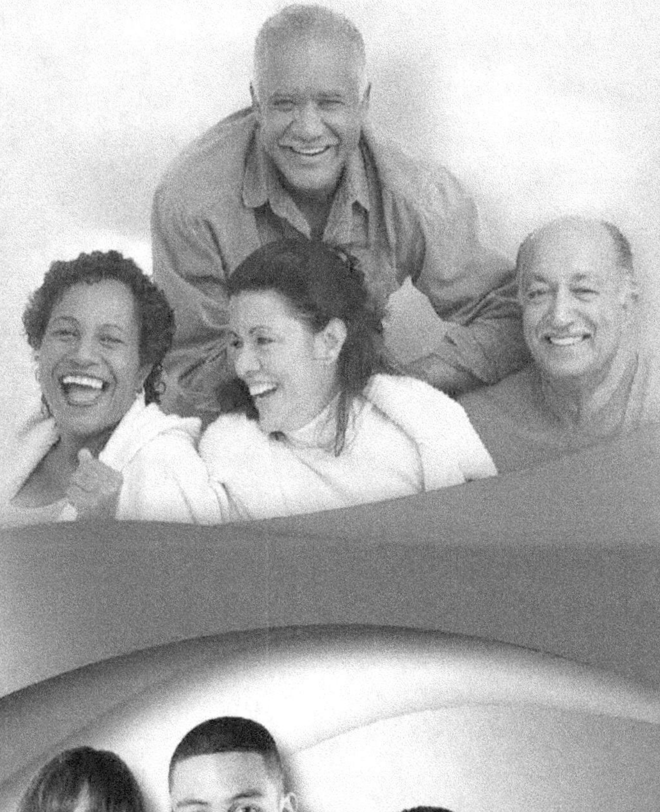

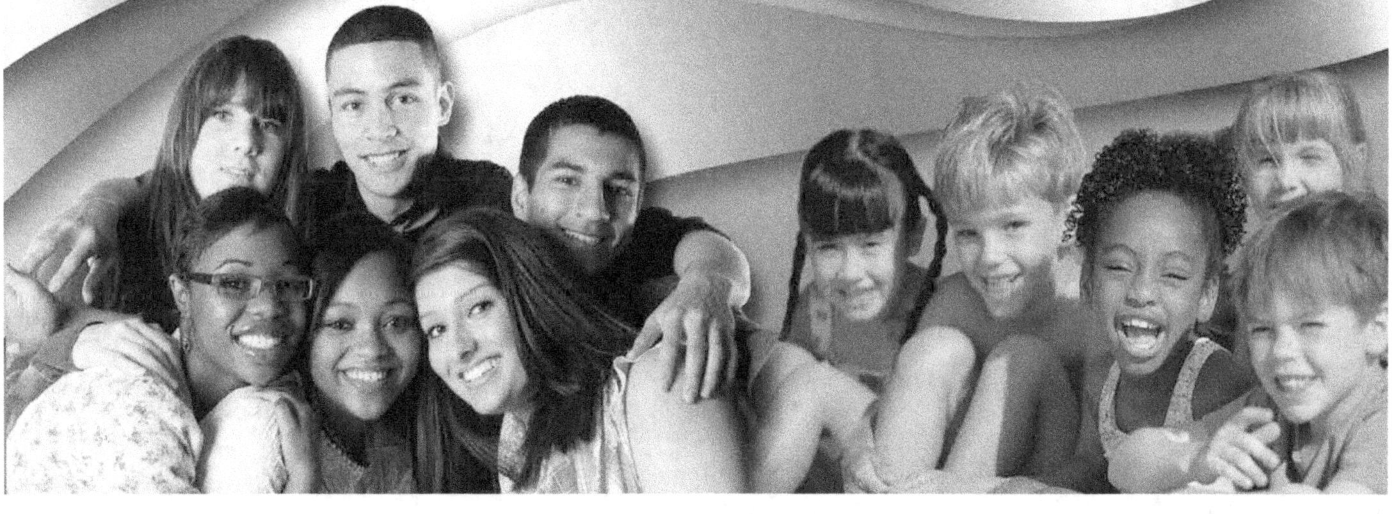

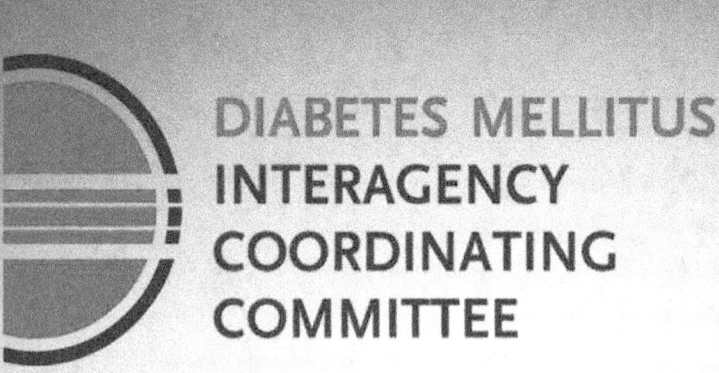

DIABETES MELLITUS
INTERAGENCY
COORDINATING
COMMITTEE

Coordinating the Federal Investment in Diabetes Programs To Improve the Health of Americans

CONTENTS

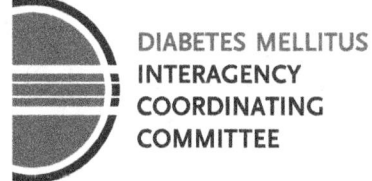

DIABETES MELLITUS
INTERAGENCY
COORDINATING
COMMITTEE

INTRODUCTION

The Diabetes Burden: Approximately 24 million people in the U.S., about 8 percent of the population, were estimated to have diabetes in 2007.[1] For the same year, diabetes cost the country an estimated $174 billion in medical expenses as well as associated costs, such as loss of workplace productivity, early disability, and morbidity.[2] The numbers reflect a striking truth: diabetes places a huge personal and economic burden on this country. However, even as rates of diabetes are rising, people with diabetes are living longer and healthier lives, as a result of the collective effort of the Diabetes Mellitus Interagency Coordinating Committee (DMICC) and others. Advances in medicine, public health, and health care have led to significant progress. New research discoveries and translation efforts will yield further improvements in the prevention, diagnosis, control, and treatment of diabetes. Building on the accomplishments and successes of federal programs in improving public health with regard to diabetes, the government agencies responsible for leading the federal investment in diabetes are working together to improve the health of Americans.

> The DMICC coordinates federal diabetes activities and works to share information, foster joint efforts, and identify opportunities for agency collaboration.

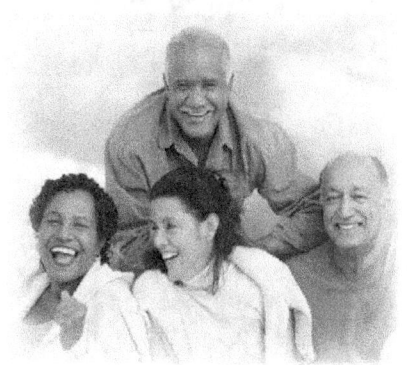

Progress Through Collaboration: Individual agencies have made significant, measurable strides in combating diabetes. However, many successful efforts have required a combination of expertise and resources not found in a single organization. The achievements highlighted in this publication exemplify what interagency coordination can accomplish when different parts of the government pull together to confront the diabetes epidemic. Such coordination is essential to avoid unnecessary duplication of diabetes activities, to maximize available resources, and to ensure the optimal use of federal funds to combat and alleviate the public health burden of diabetes.

Uniting the Federal Effort To Combat Diabetes: Congress created the statutory DMICC with the charge to coordinate diabetes research activities and health programs of the National Institutes of Health (NIH) and other federal agencies, and to provide for the communication and exchange of information necessary for coordination. The law states that the Director of the NIH, or his/her designated representative, will serve as chair of the Committee. Leadership of the Committee has been delegated to the National Institute of Diabetes and Digestive and Kidney Diseases (NIDDK).

The DMICC is uniquely positioned to leverage federal resources, minimize duplication of effort, and increase public awareness of federal diabetes research and health information.

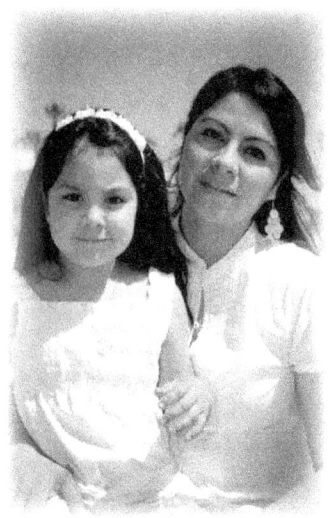

The DMICC brings together members of diverse federal agencies that conduct or support diabetes-related activities. These agencies are complementary in their missions, linking the continuum of progress toward improved diabetes outcomes, from basic research and testing of new therapies, to health care delivery and public health efforts. DMICC members include:

• The Department of Health and Human Services (DHHS): 3 Centers of the Centers for Disease Control and Prevention (CDC), 22 NIH Institutes and Centers, the Agency for Healthcare Research and Quality (AHRQ), the Centers for Medicare & Medicaid Services (CMS), the DHHS Office of Disease Prevention and Health Promotion (DHHS ODPHP), the DHHS Office of Minority Health (DHHS OMH), the Food and Drug Administration (FDA), the Health Resources and Services Administration (HRSA), and the Indian Health Service (IHS).

• Non-DHHS organizations: the Department of Defense (DOD), the U.S. Department of Agriculture (USDA), and the Veterans Health Administration (VHA).

The collaboration of DMICC member organizations has improved and will continue to improve the health of Americans.

Fostering Collaboration and Coordination: Representatives of DMICC member organizations meet in person several times annually in the Washington, D.C., area. These meetings, which bring together the top diabetes experts in the federal government, provide an opportunity for discussion of current and future projects conducted by member agencies. Presentation of projects helps members to identify opportunities for collaboration and allows them to make use of each other's expertise and resources. The meetings are incubators for the development of new ideas and projects. In addition, discussion during these meetings generates helpful input to improve ongoing programs. Meetings also serve as a forum for the planning, guidance, and evaluation of interagency initiatives.

The Future of the Federal Diabetes Effort: As the number of Americans with diabetes continues to rise, the DMICC and its members must redouble their efforts. The Committee has become a productive forum for collaboration, coordination, and pursuit of emerging opportunities. As it builds on past successes, the DMICC will embark on new efforts to advance the diabetes field by seeking novel opportunities to work together and share resources, expertise, and efforts. The members of the DMICC fully recognize that, through U.S. agency collaboration, the federal government has improved and will continue to improve the health of Americans.

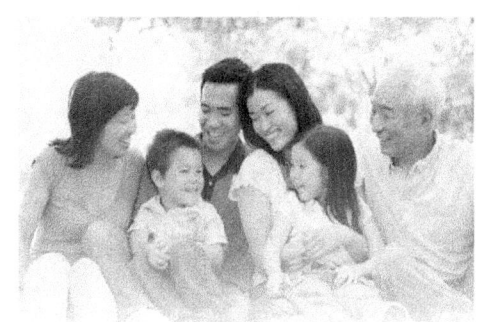

For more information about the DMICC and its activities, please visit: *http://www.diabetescommittee.gov*

What Is Gained by Coordinating Federal Diabetes-Related Efforts Through the DMICC?

- *Agencies share information and ideas.* The DMICC brings together members who are experts in diabetes and play a leading role in their respective agencies' efforts to combat the disease.

- *The DMICC fosters collaborations.* Agencies work together, combining their resources and diverse expertise to advance diabetes research and create new opportunities to improve public health.

- *Agencies translate results from research to real-world applications.* The diverse missions of DMICC member organizations span a wide range of activities, including research on diabetes, regulation of reimbursement for diabetes therapies, provision of health care, and improvement of public health. The DMICC stimulates interchange among research agencies, policymakers, and health care providers to ensure that research findings benefit the public.

Statewide Estimates of Diagnosed Diabetes (2005)

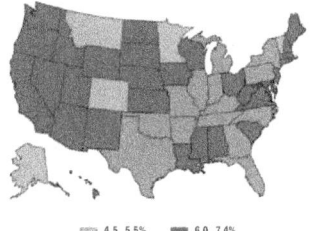

4.5 5.5%   6.0 7.4%
7.5% 8.5%   >9.0%

Figure 1. *CDC statewide estimates of diagnosed diabetes in the U.S. in 2005.* The different colors represent the percent of adults 20 years of age or older with diagnosed diabetes in 2005.[3]

County-level Estimates of Diagnosed Diabetes (2005)

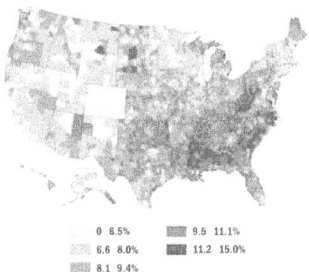

0 6.5%   9.5 11.1%
6.6 8.0%   11.2 15.0%
8.1 9.4%

Figure 2. *CDC county-level estimates of diagnosed diabetes in the U.S. in 2005.* The different colors represent the percent of adults 20 years of age or older with diagnosed diabetes in 2005.[3]

What Is Diabetes?

Diabetes is marked by high levels of blood glucose (blood sugar) resulting from defects in the production and/or action of the hormone insulin. Diabetes can lead to serious complications and premature death, but people with diabetes can take steps to control the disease and to lower the risk of complications.

Type 1 diabetes was previously called insulin-dependent diabetes mellitus or juvenile-onset diabetes. Type 1 diabetes develops when the body's immune system destroys pancreatic beta cells, the only cells in the body that make insulin. To survive, people with type 1 diabetes need insulin delivered by injection or a pump. This form of diabetes usually strikes children and young adults, although disease onset can occur at any age. In adults, type 1 diabetes accounts for 5 to 10 percent of all diagnosed cases of diabetes.[1] Risk factors for type 1 diabetes may be autoimmune, genetic, or environmental. No known way to prevent type 1 diabetes exists. Several clinical trials for the prevention of type 1 diabetes are currently in progress or are being planned.

Type 2 diabetes was previously called non-insulin-dependent diabetes mellitus or adult-onset diabetes. In adults, type 2 diabetes accounts for about 90 to 95 percent of all diagnosed cases of diabetes.[1] It usually begins as insulin resistance, a disorder in which the cells do not use insulin properly. The body reacts to this problem by producing more insulin. However, as the need for insulin rises, the pancreas gradually loses its ability to produce it. Type 2 diabetes is most often treated with medications that reduce insulin resistance and with insulin, if needed. Type 2 diabetes is associated with older age, obesity, family history of diabetes, history of gestational diabetes, impaired glucose metabolism, physical inactivity, and race/ethnicity. African Americans, Hispanic and Latino Americans, American Indians and Alaska Natives, and some Asian Americans and Native Hawaiians or other Pacific Islanders are at particularly high risk for type 2 diabetes and its complications. Type 2 diabetes in children and adolescents, although still uncommon, is being diagnosed more frequently among American Indians and Alaska Natives, African Americans, Hispanic and Latino Americans, and Asians and Pacific Islanders.

Gestational diabetes is a form of glucose intolerance diagnosed during pregnancy. Gestational diabetes occurs more frequently among African Americans, Hispanic and Latino Americans, and American Indians. It is also more common among obese women and women with a family history of diabetes. During pregnancy, gestational diabetes requires treatment to normalize maternal blood glucose levels to avoid complications in the infant. Immediately after pregnancy, 5 to 10 percent of women with gestational diabetes are found to have diabetes, usually type 2.[1] Women who have had gestational diabetes have a 40 to 60 percent chance of developing diabetes in the next 5 to 10 years.[1]

Other types of diabetes result from specific genetic conditions, such as maturity-onset diabetes of youth (MODY); surgery; medications; infections; pancreatic disease; and other illnesses. Such types of diabetes account for 1 to 5 percent of all diagnosed cases.[1]

Pre-diabetes is a condition in which blood glucose levels are higher than normal, but not as high as in diabetes. People with pre-diabetes are at high risk for developing type 2 diabetes.

Definitions of Clinical Measurements of Diabetes[4]: Several different types of tests are used by clinicians to diagnose diabetes and monitor diabetes control. The most common tests are described here.

- *Fasting blood glucose test:* In this test, blood glucose is measured after an 8-hour fast, often in the morning following an overnight fast. The fasting blood glucose test is the preferred test for diagnosing diabetes or pre-diabetes in children and nonpregnant adults.

  ▶ Normal range: 99 milligrams/deciliter (mg/dL) and below
  ▶ Range to diagnose pre-diabetes: 100 to 125 mg/dL
  ▶ Range to diagnose diabetes: 126 mg/dL and above

- *Oral glucose tolerance test:* In this test, blood glucose levels are measured after an 8-hour fast and 2 hours after an individual drinks a glucose-containing beverage. The oral glucose tolerance test can be used to diagnose diabetes or pre-diabetes, and is used to measure blood glucose levels during pregnancy.

  ▶ Normal range: 139 mg/dL and below
  ▶ Range to diagnose pre-diabetes: 140 to 199 mg/dL
  ▶ Range to diagnose diabetes: 200 mg/dL and above

- *Measurement of HbA1c Levels:* The HbA1c blood test provides information about an individual's average blood glucose levels for the past 2 to 3 months. People with diabetes should have the HbA1c test at least twice a year. The results of HbA1c tests help doctors determine whether changes in diabetes medicine, meal plans, or physical activity routine are required to keep a person's diabetes under control.

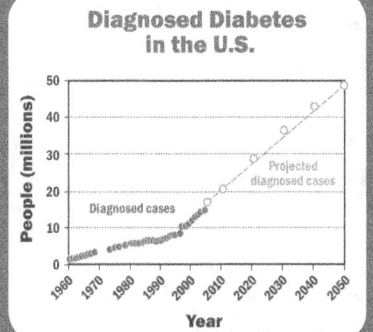

Figure 3. *Diagnosed diabetes in the U.S.* The red circles represent the number of people with diagnosed diabetes during the timeframe 1960–2004[5]; the blue circles represent the number of people who are projected to be diagnosed during the timeframe 2005–2050.[6]

The Human and Economic Toll of Diabetes in the U.S.[1,2,7]:

- As of 2007, **24 million** Americans—about 8 percent of the total population—had diabetes.

- Approximately **57 million** Americans have pre-diabetes.

- **Diabetes is the seventh** leading cause of death in the U.S.

- **One-fourth** of Americans with diabetes are undiagnosed.

- **Two-thirds** of people with diabetes die of heart disease and stroke.

- **One in three** Americans born in 2000 will develop diabetes during his or her lifetime, if current trends continue.

- The total cost attributable to diabetes for Americans was **$174 billion** in 2007, representing an increase of **32 percent** since 2002.

MEMBER ORGANIZATIONS

The DMICC is composed of representatives from 35 different federal organizations, each bringing a unique perspective and expertise to the federal diabetes effort. Even though each member has a unique role in combating the diabetes epidemic, DMICC member organizations are united in the goal of improving the health of the American people with respect to diabetes.

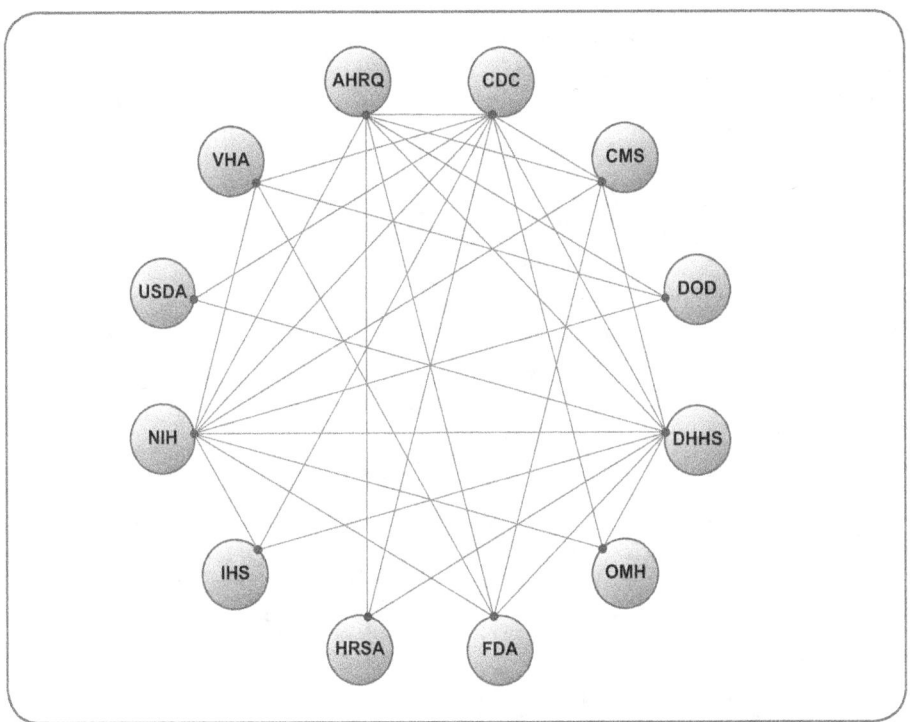

Figure 4. This graphic illustrates the interactions between DMICC member organizations on a diverse portfolio of diabetes-related activities and projects. The DMICC promotes the exchange of ideas, resources, and expertise.

Complementary Efforts To Combat Diabetes: Stopping an epidemic disease like diabetes requires simultaneous efforts on many fronts. Although all DMICC member organizations support diabetes activities, each agency's focus is unique and complementary to those of other members. This is exemplified in Figure 5, which depicts the stages of translating basic research findings to improvements in public health. The figure also shows at which steps the DMICC member organizations generally contribute to progress along the spectrum. Each of these steps requires unique resources and expertise, builds on the others, and is necessary to impact diabetes. Basic scientists seek to understand the molecular underpinnings of health and disease. In turn, this understanding yields potential targets for disease prevention and treatment that can be tested in cell and animal models (A in Figure 5).

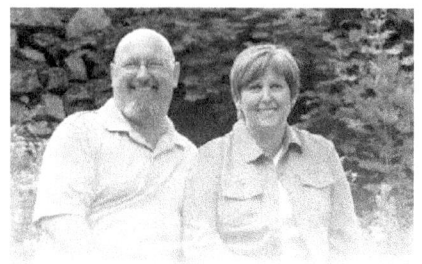

After this preclinical development, prospective interventions, whether for prevention or treatment, must be tested in humans to determine if the interventions are safe and effective. The initial testing is conducted under carefully monitored settings—at the "bedside" or in clinics under the watchful eye of clinical scientists (B). Once promising interventions are found to be beneficial in research settings, they are tested in real-world settings by investigators, translating the promise of basic research to the community (C). Often, activities that worked well in the ideal settings must be adjusted to real-world conditions.

DMICC member organizations contribute to different and complementary steps to combat diabetes.

Public health programs make interventions accessible in communities, and health care providers deliver these interventions to the people who need them (D, E). Public health officials study and monitor these interventions in the real world, evaluating which interventions have the greatest effects on the most people, and are cost-effective for public and private health care providers (E). These studies provide opportunities for collaboration among research, public health, and health care delivery organizations. The step of delivering health care is the costliest; a majority of federal spending on diabetes is used to treat people with the disease and its complications. Therefore, prevention of diabetes is critically important not only for the health of the American people, but also to reduce federal spending on diabetes care. Prevention is a high priority of federal diabetes efforts.

DMICC member organizations direct efforts in each of these steps and collaborate across steps, and together are leading the way to prevent diabetes and its complications.

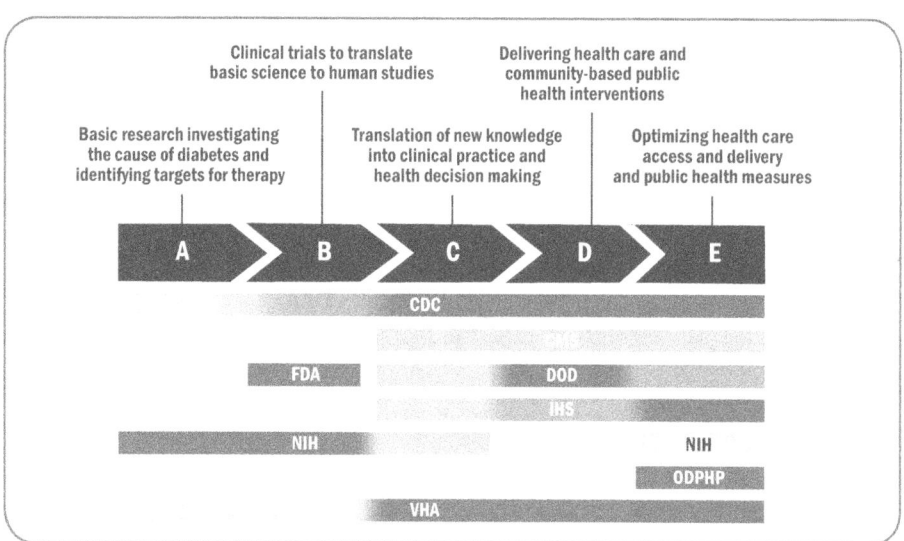

Figure 5. This graphic illustrates how DMICC member organizations are involved in different and complementary steps to combat diabetes—from understanding the underlying biology of the disease to delivering health care. The colors in the bars represent the intensity of activities at each step (from highest to lowest intensity: red, dark orange, light orange, and yellow). The intensity of activities correlates with the mission of each organization. Activities of the DMICC bring together member organizations working at these different steps to facilitate and accelerate improvements in public health.

DMICC Member Organizations

The DMICC member organizations and their missions related to diabetes are as follows:

Agency for Healthcare Research and Quality (AHRQ)
www.ahrq.gov

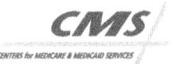 The AHRQ's mission is to improve the quality, safety, efficiency, and effectiveness of health care for all Americans. Diabetes-related programs include management of clinical guidelines in the National Guideline Clearinghouse; reports of health care quality (the National Healthcare Quality Reports and Disparities Reports); and support of comparative effectiveness studies.

Center for Scientific Review (CSR)
http://cms.csr.nih.gov

 The CSR's mission is to ensure that NIH grant applications receive fair, independent, expert, and timely reviews so that NIH can fund the most promising research. This includes the receipt, referral, and review of diabetes-related applications, and the organization of appropriate peer review study sections.

Centers for Medicare & Medicaid Services (CMS)
www.cms.hhs.gov

 CMS provides health insurance to over 40 million Medicare beneficiaries aged 65 or older or disabled. Medicare provides coverage of diabetes screening tests for beneficiaries at risk for diabetes or those diagnosed with pre-diabetes. Diabetes self-management training and medical nutrition therapy are covered services that help beneficiaries effectively manage their condition. Medicare is also testing alternative approaches to reward physicians for improving the quality and efficiency of health care delivered to beneficiaries with diabetes and other chronic conditions.

Department of Agriculture (USDA)
www.usda.gov

The USDA provides leadership on food, agriculture, natural resources, and related issues based on sound public policy, the best available science, and efficient management.

Department of Defense (DOD)
www.health.mil

The DOD's mission with respect to diabetes is to provide up-to-date, evidence-based diabetic care to all DOD beneficiaries. Diabetes-related programs include the development and publication of clinical practice guidelines, in collaboration with VHA, and investigations to improve the cost-effectiveness and efficiency of care.

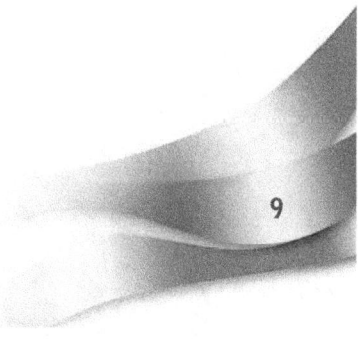

Department of Health and Human Services Office of Disease Prevention and Health Promotion (DHHS ODPHP)
www.odphp.osophs.dhhs.gov

 The DHHS ODPHP's mission is to provide leadership for a healthier America by initiating, coordinating, and supporting disease prevention and health promotion programs, policies, and information. Diabetes-related programs include development of *Healthy People 2010*, a nationwide health promotion and disease prevention agenda; review of dietary guidance materials; coordination of departmental responses on nutrition; and management of *www.healthfinder.gov* to link consumers and professionals to more than 6,000 resources from the federal government and its partners.

Department of Health and Human Services Office of Minority Health (DHHS OMH)
www.omhrc.gov

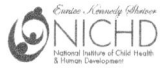 The DHHS OMH's mission is to improve and protect the health of racial and ethnic minority populations through the development of health policies and programs that will eliminate health disparities.

Eunice Kennedy Shriver National Institute of Child Health and Human Development (NICHD)
www.nichd.nih.gov

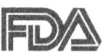 The NICHD's mission is to promote the development of healthy children. Toward this goal, NICHD conducts and supports diabetes-related research, including efforts to understand the genetic and environmental factors that contribute to the development of diabetes, to elucidate the earliest symptoms of type 1 diabetes and the precursors of type 2 diabetes, to improve the outcome of pregnancy in women with gestational diabetes, and to optimize insulin therapy in children with type 1 diabetes.

Food and Drug Administration (FDA)
www.fda.gov

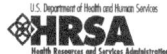 The FDA's mission is to ensure the availability of safe and effective therapies in the management of diabetes by providing guidance and oversight of clinical development of drugs and biologics.

Health Resources and Services Administration (HRSA)
www.hrsa.gov

 The HRSA provides national leadership, program resources, and services needed to improve access to culturally competent, quality health care.

Indian Health Service (IHS)
www.ihs.gov

The mission of IHS is to raise the physical, mental, social, and spiritual health of American Indians and Alaska Natives to the highest levels. The mission of the IHS Division of Diabetes Treatment and Prevention is to develop, document, and sustain a public health effort to prevent and control diabetes in American Indians and Alaska Native peoples.

National Center for Chronic Disease Prevention and Health Promotion (NCCDPHP)
www.cdc.gov/diabetes

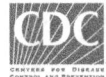 The mission of CDC's Division of Diabetes Translation (DDT) within NCCDPHP is to reduce the preventable burden of diabetes through public health leadership, partnerships, research, programs, and policies that translate science into practice. The Division's main focus is to achieve the greatest impact for populations with the greatest burden or risk through surveillance, translational research, and state, territorial, and tribal-based Diabetes Prevention and Control Programs, and national wellness and education programs.

National Center for Complementary and Alternative Medicine (NCCAM)
www.nccam.nih.gov

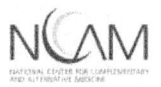 The NCCAM's mission is to investigate the basic and clinical use of complementary and alternative therapies, including therapies for the treatment of diabetes and related complications. Diabetes-related programs include support for research on chromium treatment of obesity-related insulin resistance, fatty acid supplementation in people with type 2 diabetes, and the effects of fish oil and related compounds on the progression of insulin resistance.

National Center for Environmental Health (NCEH)
www.cdc.gov/nceh/dls

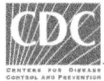 The mission of CDC's Division of Laboratory Sciences within NCEH is to improve and standardize laboratory measurement of biomarkers for assessing diabetes risk and for monitoring treatment and disease status.

National Center for Health Statistics (NCHS)
www.cdc.gov/nchs

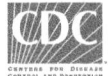 The mission of CDC NCHS is to compile statistical information to guide actions and policies to improve health. NCHS collects data from birth and death records, medical records, interview surveys, and through direct physical exams and laboratory testing. These national data systems provide diabetes-related information for public health efforts to reduce the impact of diabetes.

National Center for Research Resources (NCRR)
www.ncrr.nih.gov

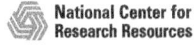 The NCRR's mission is to provide clinical and translational researchers with the training and tools to transform basic discoveries into improved human health. NCRR leads NIH's Clinical and Translational Science Award (CTSA) program to create a definable academic home for the discipline of clinical and translational science at institutions across the country. The CTSA program will foster clinical research on diabetes and its complications. In addition, NCRR collaborated with NIDDK to support an aggressive program in supporting islet cell research by providing viable, isolated islets to NIH-approved investigators. NCRR participated in the transfer of this support to NIDDK in 2009.

National Center on Minority Health and Health Disparities (NCMHD)
www.ncmhd.nih.gov

 The NCMHD's mission is to promote minority health, and to lead, coordinate, support, and assess the NIH's effort to reduce and ultimately eliminate health disparities.

National Eye Institute (NEI)
www.nei.nih.gov

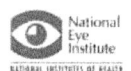 The NEI's mission is to conduct and support vision research, training, health information dissemination, and programs, including the detection, treatment, and prevention of diabetic eye disease. NEI supports and oversees the Diabetic Retinopathy Clinical Research Network and coordinates the National Eye Health Education Program to raise awareness and to educate on the importance of early detection and timely treatment of diabetic eye disease.

National Heart, Lung, and Blood Institute (NHLBI)
www.nhlbi.nih.gov

The NHLBI's mission is to provide leadership for a national program in diseases of the heart, blood vessels, lung, and blood; blood resources; and sleep disorders. Because diabetes is a major risk factor for heart disease, NHLBI is committed to supporting research to understand, treat, and prevent the link between diabetes and its vascular complications. Diabetes-related programs include clinical trials examining intervention strategies in populations with diabetes and pre-diabetes.

National Human Genome Research Institute (NHGRI)
www.genome.gov

 Since leading NIH's contribution to the International Human Genome Project, NHGRI has expanded its mission to encompass a broad range of studies aimed at understanding the structure and function of the human genome and its role in health and disease. Diabetes-related programs include the genetic analysis of traits related to type 2 diabetes, programs on clinical integration and health disparities of type 2 diabetes, and studies related to the implications of genetic and genomic research.

National Institute on Aging (NIA)
www.nia.nih.gov

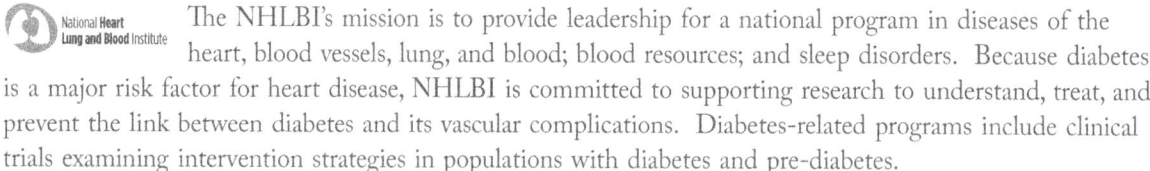 The NIA's mission is to improve the health and well-being of older Americans through research, with a goal of developing safe and effective treatment approaches for elderly people with diabetes. Diabetes-related programs include research to: understand the relationships among obesity, insulin signaling, hypertension, and diabetes; study the efficacy of approaches to maintain a healthy weight and prevent diabetes; determine whether recommendations for healthy eating, physical exercise, and sleep are optimal for older people; and elucidate the causes of disparities in the prevalence of obesity and diabetes among minority and underserved populations.

National Institute on Alcohol Abuse and Alcoholism (NIAAA)
www.niaaa.nih.gov

 The NIAAA provides leadership in the national effort to reduce alcohol-related problems by conducting and supporting research in a wide range of scientific areas; coordinating and collaborating with other research institutes, federal programs, institutions, organizations, agencies, and programs on alcohol-related issues; and translating and disseminating research findings to health care providers, researchers, policymakers, and the public.

National Institute of Allergy and Infectious Diseases (NIAID)
www3.niaid.nih.gov

 The NIAID conducts and supports basic and applied research to better understand, treat, and ultimately prevent infectious, immunologic, and allergic diseases.

National Institute of Biomedical Imaging and Bioengineering (NIBIB)
www.nibib.nih.gov

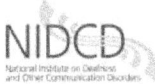 The NIBIB's mission is to improve health by promoting fundamental discoveries and translation of technological capabilities in biomedical imaging and bioengineering. Diabetes-related programs include efforts to develop novel approaches to image beta cells and their function in normal and diseased pancreas and transplanted islets; and to develop tissue engineering/regenerative medicine, drug and gene delivery, and medical implant technologies for diabetes.

National Institute on Deafness and Other Communication Disorders (NIDCD)
www.nidcd.nih.gov

The NIDCD's mission is to conduct and support biomedical and behavioral research in the normal and disordered processes of hearing, balance, smell, taste, voice, speech, and language. Individuals with smell and taste disorders can become obese and develop diabetes, so research in this field could be important to the prevention of diabetes. Recently, NIDCD investigators determined that hearing loss is twice as common in adults with diabetes as in those who do not have the disease, highlighting the importance of research on the relationship between diabetes and hearing.

National Institute of Dental and Craniofacial Research (NIDCR)
www.nidcr.nih.gov/OralHealth/Topics/Diabetes

The NIDCR's mission is to improve oral, dental, and craniofacial health through research, research training, and dissemination of health information. The NIDCR supports basic and clinical research to define the relationship between diabetes and oral health. For example, people with diabetes are at increased risk for gum disease. Current diabetes-related programs include a Phase III clinical trial to test whether treatment of gum disease improves glycemic control in patients with type 2 diabetes, and research to examine the oral health of children with type 1 diabetes.

National Institute of Diabetes and Digestive and Kidney Diseases (NIDDK)
www2.niddk.nih.gov

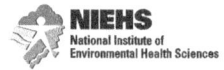 The NIDDK's mission with respect to diabetes is to conduct and support basic, clinical, and translational research to improve the understanding, treatment, and prevention of the disease and its complications. The NIDDK, on behalf of the Secretary of DHHS, oversees the *Special Statutory Funding Program for Type 1 Diabetes Research* on the prevention of and cure for type 1 diabetes. The mission of NIDDK also includes extending the benefits of research to the public through provision of public health information.

National Institute on Drug Abuse (NIDA)
www.nida.nih.gov

 The NIDA's mission is to support research on basic, epidemiological, clinical, and translational aspects of drug abuse and comorbid conditions, including infections. NIDA supports research on endocrine, gastrointestinal, and metabolic disorders, including diabetes, in their relation to infections such as HIV and hepatitis C, or to antiretroviral therapy in substance-abusing patients.

National Institute of Environmental Health Sciences (NIEHS)
www.niehs.nih.gov

 The NIEHS' mission is to reduce the burden of human illness and disability by understanding how the environment influences the development and progression of human disease.

National Institute of General Medical Sciences (NIGMS)
www.nigms.nih.gov

The NIGMS' mission is to support research that increases the understanding of life processes and lays the foundation for advances in disease diagnosis, treatment, and prevention. The NIGMS funds research to investigate the basic science of health and disease, including diabetes.

National Institute of Mental Health (NIMH)
www.nimh.nih.gov

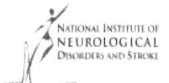 The NIMH's mission is to transform the understanding and treatment of mental illnesses through basic and clinical research, paving the way for prevention, recovery, and cure.

National Institute of Neurological Disorders and Stroke (NINDS)
www.ninds.nih.gov

The NINDS' mission is to reduce the burden of neurological disease that is borne by every age group, by every segment of society, and by people all over the world.

National Institute of Nursing Research (NINR)
www.ninr.nih.gov

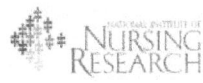 The NINR's mission is to support basic and clinical research to establish a scientific basis for the care of individuals across the lifespan; it focuses on all those affected by diabetes—from individuals, to families, to caregivers—with a special emphasis on the needs of underserved populations. The NINR supports a broad range of research, from the genetic and biobehavioral mechanisms underlying the development of diabetes to age-appropriate and community-oriented interventions to prevent and manage diabetes symptoms and complications.

National Library of Medicine (NLM)
www.nlm.nih.gov

 The NLM's mission is to collect, organize, and disseminate information on all areas of biomedicine and health care, including diabetes, using the latest informatics tools and strategies. The NLM maintains electronic resources for both scientists and the public, including Web sites (*http://MedlinePlus. gov, http://ClinicalTrials.gov*), databases (PubMed®, MEDLINE®), and the resources of the National Center for Biotechnology Information.

Veterans Health Administration (VHA)
www1.va.gov/diabetes/index.cfm

 The mission of the VHA diabetes program is to improve the health of veterans at risk for or with diabetes by decreasing the incidence of adverse health outcomes. This is achieved through systems-level integration of evidence-based clinical practice guidelines, performance measurements, data feedback, and education to promote the increased use of evidence-based preventative and treatment processes. The VHA research service supports this mission through basic, clinical, and health services research.

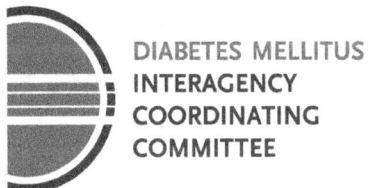

DIABETES MELLITUS
INTERAGENCY
COORDINATING
COMMITTEE

EXAMPLES OF COORDINATION OF FEDERAL DIABETES ACTIVITIES

Creation and Support of the National Diabetes Education Program

Research-Based Diabetes Health Campaigns: The National Diabetes Education Program (NDEP) was launched in 1997 to improve diabetes control and to reduce the morbidity and mortality associated with diabetes complications. The initial campaign was built on the findings of NIDDK's landmark Diabetes Control and Complications Trial (DCCT), which demonstrated that keeping blood glucose levels as close to normal as possible slows the onset and progression of the eye, kidney, and nerve damage caused by diabetes. After the Diabetes Prevention Program (DPP) clinical trial proved that delay or prevention of type 2 diabetes is possible (see next section), the NDEP expanded its focus to diabetes prevention.

> The DMICC provides input to the NDEP for translating the latest science and spreading the word that diabetes is serious, common, and costly, yet *controllable* or *preventable*.

Recommended by the National Diabetes Advisory Board, the NDEP is the leading federal government public education program that promotes diabetes prevention and control. DMICC member organizations not only contribute to the development and distribution of NDEP materials, but many members also participate as federal agency liaisons to NDEP's Coordinating Committee. The program's oversight and sponsorship—by NIDDK and CDC DDT—provides a firm basis of credibility, commitment, resources, and connections to federal, state, and local public health agencies nationwide.

NDEP products, resources, and tools are available at www.ndep. nih.gov

The NDEP develops and disseminates products, resources, and tools for local, state, and national distribution. These tools and resources are intended for multiple audiences, such as people with diabetes and their families, including children; populations at high risk for diabetes; health care professionals; payers and purchasers of health care; health care system policymakers; and business professionals. NDEP's partnerships with more than 200 health professional, community, consumer, and private sector organizations ensure broad and meaningful input in design, effective implementation, and wide dissemination of messages and educational tools.

Major NDEP Campaigns Target Diabetes Prevention and Control: To help address health disparities and meet the goals of the major federal government public health initiative titled *Healthy People 2010*, the NDEP developed two major campaigns based on scientific studies of diabetes prevention and control:

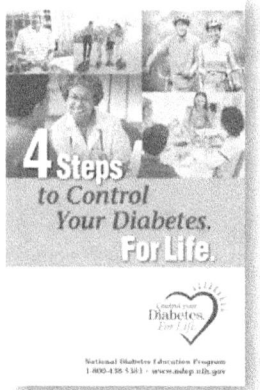

- **Control Your Diabetes. For Life:** This campaign promotes the importance of comprehensive diabetes control. Initially based on findings from DCCT, and subsequently expanded to include findings from clinical trials worldwide, the campaign has distilled essential information into easy-to-read materials for people with diabetes and their loved ones, and for the health care team. Campaign materials present the message that comprehensive control is the key to preventing heart attack and stroke, which kill two out of every three people with diabetes, as well as in preventing blindness, amputation, and kidney failure. The campaign highlights the ABCs of diabetes control: *A* for the HbA1c test to measure blood glucose control, *B* for blood pressure, and *C* for cholesterol. For more information, visit: *www.ndep.nih.gov/campaigns/ControlForLife/ControlForLife_overview.htm*

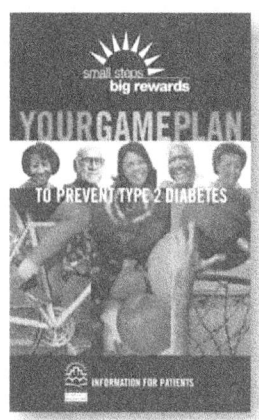

- **Small Steps. Big Rewards. Prevent Type 2 Diabetes:** The nation's first comprehensive multicultural diabetes prevention campaign, *Small Steps. Big Rewards. Prevent type 2 Diabetes.* is intended to stem the diabetes epidemic by targeting the 57 million Americans with pre-diabetes.[1] Based on the groundbreaking findings from the DPP clinical trial, the campaign delivers practical, real-world tools to help people take the small steps needed to achieve the big reward of preventing or delaying type 2 diabetes. Messages and materials have been tailored and adapted for groups at high risk for type 2 diabetes, including African Americans, American Indians, Alaska Natives, Asian Americans, Hispanic and Latino Americans, Pacific Islanders, older adults, and women with a history of gestational diabetes. For more information, visit: *www.ndep.nih.gov/campaigns/SmallSteps/SmallSteps_overview.htm*

The NDEP is committed to evaluating its programs and to assessing its value in improving the health of people with diabetes and people at risk for the disease. This enables the program to gain new insights for planning and implementation strategies, and to continually refine its efforts to deliver crucial health messages. The NDEP also is continually updating and adapting its messages as new information becomes available. For example, in 2008, the results of several diabetes clinical trials suggested that a "one-size-fits-all" approach to diabetes treatment may not be the

> In 2007 alone, more than 221 million pairs of "eyes and ears" saw, heard, or read NDEP messages on television and radio, and in print and online newspapers and magazines.

best way to care for patients. One of those trials was Action to Control Cardiovascular Risk in Diabetes (ACCORD), which is led by NHLBI with support from NIDDK, NIA, NEI, and CDC DDT. ACCORD studied older patients with longstanding diabetes and with or at very high risk for cardiovascular disease, and found that intensive metabolic control—aiming for HbA1c goals below the American Diabetes Association (ADA) guidelines—could increase risk of death. To include information from this and other important trials, the NDEP is modulating its message: ADA guidelines for HbA1c level goals are still appropriate, but patients need to talk to their doctors and may need to develop individualized target levels.

It Takes a Community—The NDEP Reaches Out To Get Everyone Involved:
Although the NDEP has a national focus, it also seeks to reach people at the community level—where we live, work, worship, and play. The NDEP strives to ensure that community organizations have the means, knowledge, and resources to best serve their communities. To help organizations reduce the burden of diabetes among high-risk populations at the community level, the NDEP, through a competitive process, awards funding to national organizations. Examples of resulting community resources follow.

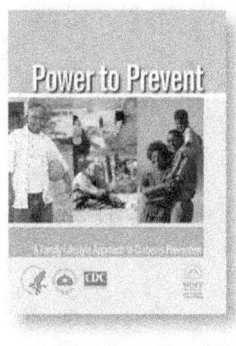

- *Power to Prevent: A Family Lifestyle Approach to Diabetes Prevention* is a culturally relevant program for African American communities about diabetes prevention and control through healthy eating and physical activity. More information is available at: *www.ndep.nih.gov/diabetes/pubs/power-to-prevent.pdf*

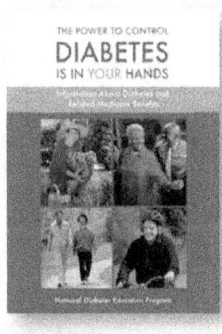

- *The Power to Control Diabetes Is in Your Hands Community Outreach Kit* is an online resource with information about diabetes in older adults and the importance of comprehensive diabetes control. More information is available at: *www.ndep.nih.gov/diabetes/pubs/Power_Comm_Kit.pdf*

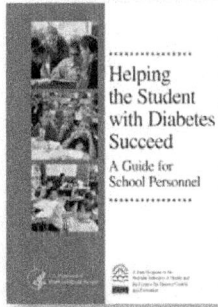

- *Helping the Student with Diabetes Succeed: A Guide for School Personnel* is a comprehensive guide that provides school personnel, parents, and students with a framework for managing diabetes effectively in the school setting. More information is available at: *www.ndep.nih.gov/diabetes/pubs/Youth_NDEPSchoolGuide.pdf*

DMICC member organizations distribute NDEP materials through their Web sites or in print to raise awareness about diabetes prevention and management.

How Do DMICC Member Organizations Utilize the NDEP To Achieve Their Missions?

DMICC members collaborate on NDEP activities and use NDEP materials to benefit the people they serve.

Collaborations with the NDEP: Several DMICC member organizations collaborate with the NDEP. For example, IHS has worked with the NDEP to develop materials specific to American Indian and Alaska Native populations, including the *We Have the Power to Prevent Diabetes* campaign. The VHA has collaborated with the NDEP in multiple ways, such as inviting the NDEP to present at an annual meeting and partnering with the NDEP on the *Feet Can Last a Lifetime* kit.

Distribution of NDEP materials at events: DMICC members distribute NDEP materials at education and outreach events. For example, the Kentucky Diabetes Prevention and Control Program, sponsored by CDC DDT, conducted a wellness program at a local worksite. More than 1,000 employees received onsite training to promote better diabetes control and prevention using NDEP campaign materials. Efforts are ongoing to expand this program to other worksites in the U.S.

Direction to the NDEP Web site: Many DMICC member organizations choose to provide links to the NDEP through their respective Web sites. This ensures that online visitors seeking diabetes health information are directed to these important and useful resources. For example, both *www.healthfinder.gov*, a health information Web site coordinated by DHHS ODPHP, and *http://MedlinePlus.gov*, an online medical resource overseen by NLM, link to the NDEP Web site. The VHA's Veterans Affairs Diabetes Program homepage also directs visitors to the NDEP Web site.

Links to specific NDEP materials: DMICC member organizations also provide online links to NDEP materials that relate specifically to their respective missions. For example, NIDCR's Web site links to the brochure *Working Together to Manage Diabetes: A Guide for Pharmacy, Podiatry, Optometry, and Dental Professionals*.

Staff education: DMICC member organizations use NDEP materials internally to provide their staff with up-to-date, clear, consistent information. For example, AHRQ distributes materials within its organization.

Information for scientists and health care professionals: NDEP materials are used by DMICC member organizations to educate researchers and health care providers. For example, NIDA shares NDEP materials with investigators interested in pursuing research related to diabetes, and VHA distributes NDEP materials to diabetes educators.

Coordinating Federal Efforts To Prevent Type 2 Diabetes

Diabetes rates are rising nationwide in all ages and ethnic groups. To combat this trend, NIDDK and its collaborators launched the Diabetes Prevention Program (DPP) clinical trial to test whether type 2 diabetes could be prevented or delayed in overweight people with blood glucose levels that were higher than normal. The trial, conducted between 1995 and 2001, compared three approaches to prevent diabetes: standard medical advice about diet and exercise, intensive lifestyles changes aimed at achieving a 5 to 7 percent weight loss through diet and moderate exercise, and treatment with the diabetes drug metformin. The DPP demonstrated that lifestyle changes that led to modest weight loss reduced the onset of type 2 diabetes by a dramatic 58 percent. Treatment with the diabetes drug metformin reduced diabetes risk by 31 percent. The interventions worked in all ethnic and racial groups studied and in both men and women. Because of the trial's collaborative nature—and because its findings would impact the activities of all federal agencies involved in diabetes—the results of this landmark clinical trial were announced by then-DHHS Secretary Tommy Thompson at a meeting of the DMICC. Since the announcement of these landmark results, DMICC member organizations have made prevention of diabetes a high priority.

> The results of the landmark DPP, which dramatically showed that type 2 diabetes can be prevented or delayed, were announced by then-DHHS Secretary Tommy Thompson at the August 2001 meeting of the DMICC. Prevention of diabetes is a high priority of federal diabetes efforts.

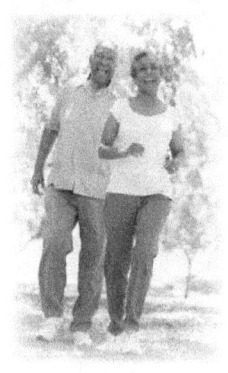

DPP Collaborations Lead to a Landmark Trial in Diabetes Prevention: Led by NIDDK, the DPP was supported by many collaborators, including NIA, NEI, NICHD, NCMHD, NIH Office of Research on Women's Health, NIH Office of Behavioral and Social Sciences Research, CDC DDT, and IHS. Coordination and collaboration informed the overall design of the trial. The CDC's population-wide data showed that rates of type 2 diabetes were very high in older people and minority populations.[1] Therefore, NIDDK designed the trial so that 45 percent of the participants were from minority groups. The IHS was instrumental in involving the participation of American Indians—a population with the highest rates of diabetes in the country.[1] A significant number of DPP participants were over age 60; funding provided by NIA enabled their inclusion.

Other DMICC collaborators played critical roles in the DPP. For example, support from the NIH Office of Research on Women's Health and NICHD facilitated the inclusion in the trial of women with gestational diabetes. The CDC DDT supported measurement and analysis of the cost-effectiveness of the interventions, which is critically important for implementing nationwide health care efforts. Support from NHLBI provided for the assessment of complications in the follow-up study to the DPP, the Diabetes Prevention Program Outcomes Study (DPPOS). The DPPOS

The design and conduct of the DPP were beyond the scope, resources, and expertise of any one government agency. Together, the collaborators effectively designed and conducted a landmark clinical trial that changed the approach to type 2 diabetes prevention in the U.S.

21

is studying the long-term effect of diet and exercise and metformin on the delay of type 2 diabetes in participants of the DPP. Finally, the private sector also provided support for the DPP.

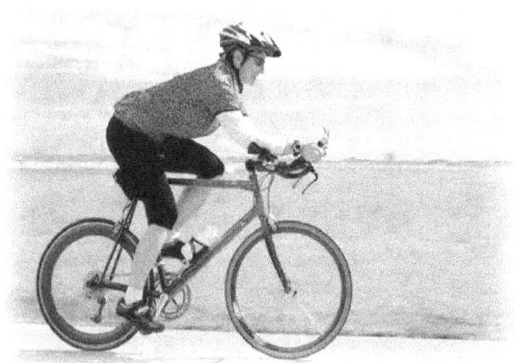

Translating the DPP Findings To Help People:
DMICC member organizations are working together to spread the word to the American people about preventing type 2 diabetes. Since the DPP results were announced, several DMICC meetings have focused on the best ways to translate the findings. The DMICC meetings facilitate the sharing of information and provide a forum for discussion of how best to work together to use the DPP results to improve public health. Examples of how DMICC members coordinate efforts follow.

- The DPP findings informed the creation of a new campaign of the NDEP, *Small Steps. Big Rewards. Prevent type 2 Diabetes*. The nation's first comprehensive, multicultural, diabetes educational campaign emphasizes the effectiveness of a healthier lifestyle in preventing the disease. DMICC member organizations use *Small Steps* campaign materials in their education and outreach efforts. For example, IHS uses materials tailored to American Indians and Alaska Natives to help this high-risk population prevent type 2 diabetes. In addition, CDC DDT-funded state-based Diabetes Prevention and Control Programs have launched local billboard, radio, print, and television campaigns using *Small Steps* materials.

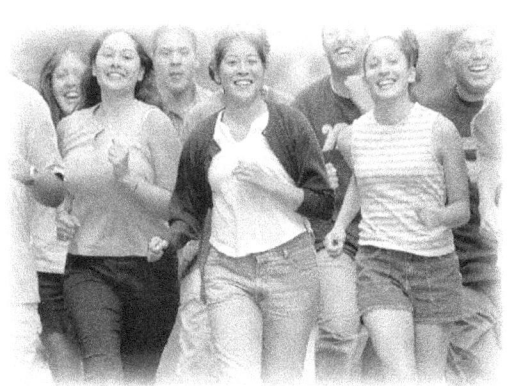

- The NIDDK and CDC DDT support translational research efforts to find ways to implement the DPP lifestyle intervention in real-world settings. For example, complementary studies funded by NIDDK and CDC DDT are examining the feasibility of using the YMCA system to deliver a DPP lifestyle intervention. Through the DMICC, NIDDK and CDC DDT share the results of similar studies with federal agencies and external organizations that deliver health care and support community outreach, to ensure that successful approaches are broadly implemented to help the American people.

• Building upon lessons learned from the DPP, CDC DDT established the Diabetes Primary Prevention Initiative. The initiative is a collaboration with AHRQ, state-based Diabetes Prevention and Control Programs, and national organizations that identifies strategies for federal, state, and local public health implementation of diabetes primary prevention. In 2005, CDC DDT initiated several statewide pilot programs to explore type 2 diabetes primary prevention in the areas of interventions, surveillance, and system dynamics modeling. Lessons learned from the initiative will be shared to increase opportunities for implementation at the local level.

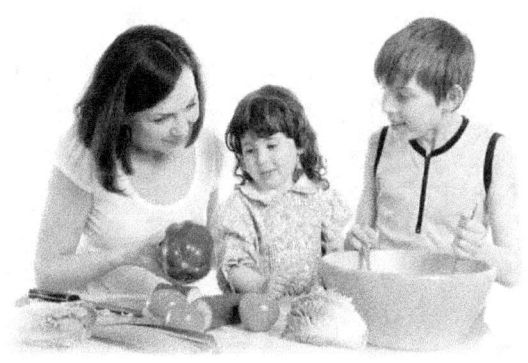

DPP Interventions Are Cost-Effective: The DPP clearly showed that type 2 diabetes can be prevented or delayed. Because so many people have pre-diabetes, are these interventions cost-effective to the U.S. health care system? To find out, CDC DDT supported a cost-effectiveness analysis and estimated that the DPP lifestyle intervention would cost society about $8,800 per "quality-adjusted life year," and the metformin intervention would cost society about $29,900 per "quality-adjusted life year" saved over the lifetime of a patient. These costs are within the range typically acceptable for health care interventions. This analysis was important to demonstrate that the interventions are affordable on a nationwide scale.

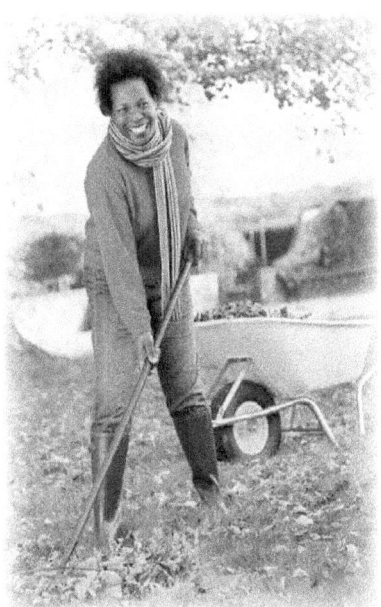

DMICC Looks to the Future: Diabetes prevention is the underpinning of any effort to curb the diabetes epidemic. In many ways, the DPP's encouraging results can be viewed as an initial step in the path toward prevention. However, much work remains to be done. The DMICC has assumed the critical responsibility of coordinating efforts to educate and empower individuals, communities, and systems that will support prevention of type 2 diabetes. The DMICC also is ensuring that strategies to implement the DPP in real-world settings are broadly disseminated to the people who can benefit most from them. DMICC members are committed to working together to make diabetes prevention a reality, thus sparing people from a relentless, debilitating disease, and improving public health.

Combating Diabetes in Communities

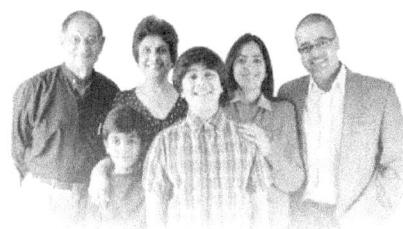

The DMICC Coordinates Efforts To Address Diabetes in Special Populations: Type 1 and type 2 diabetes do not discriminate based on age, race, ethnicity, or gender—diabetes can affect any person at any time. However, certain racial and ethnic populations are more frequently affected by diabetes. The DMICC actively coordinates federal efforts to combat the diabetes epidemic in special populations. Several DMICC meetings have focused on this topic and have served to synergize federal efforts. For example, a DMICC meeting on "approaches integrating epidemiological data on diabetes" focused on how best to use population-wide information about diabetes. Members discussed ways to use these data to understand the obstacles to screening and predicting disease risk in specific populations. Such meetings help foster collaboration, information-sharing, and efforts to reduce overlap in federal programs.

> **The DMICC actively coordinates federal efforts to address the diabetes epidemic in special populations.**

DMICC member organizations collaborate with the NDEP, which tailors culturally appropriate diabetes education materials to groups at highest risk for diabetes. Many NDEP materials are available in multiple languages, from Spanish to Samoan, to ensure that prevention materials reach as many people as possible. The NDEP also develops educational materials for older adults, women with a history of gestational diabetes, and children and teenagers. The reach of NDEP's public education campaigns has been extensive and includes the worksite and health care settings.

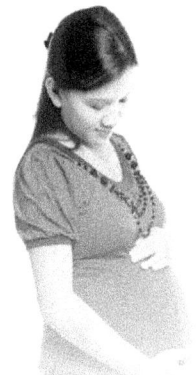

Special Populations Affected by Diabetes

Minority groups: Type 2 diabetes occurs more frequently among minority groups, including African Americans, Hispanic and Latino Americans, American Indians, Alaska Natives, Asian Americans, and Pacific Islanders.

Older Americans: The CDC estimates that nearly 25 percent of people age 60 and older in the U.S. have diabetes.[i] For older people with diabetes, the disease often limits their ability to function normally.

Women of childbearing age: Women may develop gestational diabetes during pregnancy, which can harm their offspring and increase the mothers' and children's chances of developing type 2 diabetes in the future. Babies born to mothers with pre-existing diabetes (e.g., type 1 or type 2 diabetes) are healthier if diabetes is well-controlled prior to conception and during pregnancy.

Children and adolescents: Type 1 diabetes is usually diagnosed in infancy, childhood, adolescence, or young adulthood. As a result of increased overweight and obesity, type 2 diabetes is increasingly being diagnosed in children and adolescents, particularly in minority youth. Managing diabetes is an enormous burden for both parents and the children.

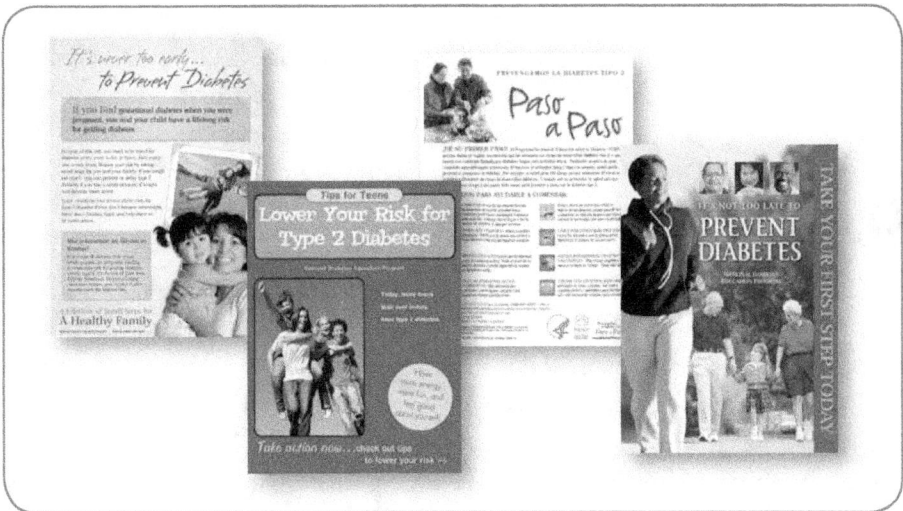

Figure 6. Co-led by NIH and CDC DDT, NDEP tailors educational materials for special populations such as women with a history of gestational diabetes, teenagers, minorities, and older people.

Improving the Health of Hispanic and Latino Communities:

Two and a half million Hispanics and Latinos in the U.S. (almost 10 percent) age 20 years or older have diabetes, and nearly 50 percent of all Hispanic and Latino children are projected to develop diabetes at some point during their lifetimes, according to CDC estimates.[1, 3] These are frightening statistics and predictions, but there is hope, because diabetes can be controlled and even delayed or prevented. DMICC member organizations are involved in numerous efforts to improve the health of Hispanic and Latino communities. For

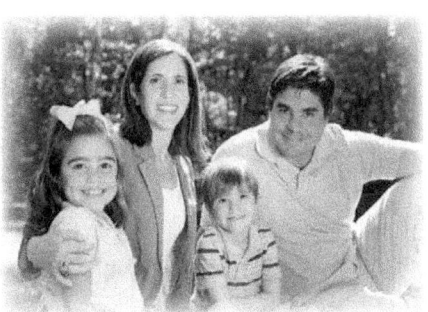

example, AHRQ, CDC DDT, CMS, and HRSA are collaborating to assist communities in developing coordinated strategies for improving the health of elderly Hispanics. The Hispanic Elders Initiative brings together teams of local leaders from communities with large numbers of Hispanic elders to learn about advances in research and clinical practice, and to receive assistance in using this information to create and implement their own local plans. This project emphasizes the importance of working across organizational boundaries to unite service providers for the elderly, medical care providers, Hispanic community organizations, and public agencies to reduce health disparities within this population.

DMICC member organizations also are analyzing the utility of health information materials for these communities. The NLM conducts and supports outreach projects with special populations, particularly underrepresented minorities, to demonstrate and evaluate the utility of electronic health information resources. For example, NLM supports an ongoing study to determine whether Hispanic and Latino people with diabetes benefit from accessing *http://MedlinePlus.gov* for health information.

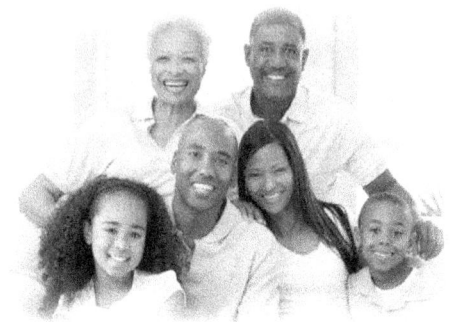

Fighting Diabetes in African American Communities:
The CDC estimates that 3.7 million (about 15 percent) of all non-Hispanic blacks age 20 years and older have diagnosed or undiagnosed diabetes.[1] DMICC member organizations are working together to support research in this population, to develop tailored outreach materials, and to improve the delivery and quality of health care. For example, DMICC members are using materials developed by NIDDK, in collaboration with CDC DDT, to highlight the importance of accurate methods to measure HbA1c levels in people with diabetes who also have sickle cell trait or other inherited forms of variant hemoglobin. People of African, Mediterranean, or Southeast Asian heritage are more likely to have a hemoglobin variant. Some clinical laboratory methods to measure HbA1c yield unreliable results in patients with sickle cell trait. Inaccurate HbA1c readings, whether falsely high or low, may lead to the over-treatment or under-treatment of diabetes. The specific needs for testing blood glucose control in these patients are explained in two booklets available from NIDDK's National Diabetes Information Clearinghouse, one for patients (*http://diabetes.niddk.nih.gov/dm/pubs/traitA1C/index.htm*) and one for physicians (*http://diabetes.niddk.nih.gov/dm/pubs/hemovari-A1C/index.htm*).

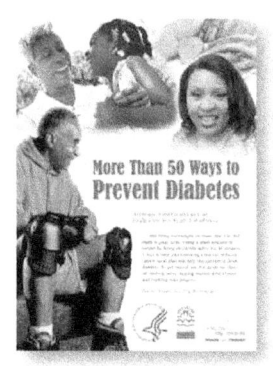

The NDEP has tailored resources to help African American families lower their risk for type 2 diabetes. The NDEP developed a diabetes prevention campaign around a "family reunion" theme highlighting the importance of learning whether diabetes runs in the family. *Ten Ways to Shape Up Your Family Reunion to Prevent Type 2 Diabetes* includes practical tips for African Americans and their families on losing weight by making healthy food choices and incorporating more physical activity into family reunions. More information is available at: *www.ndep.nih.gov/diabetes/pubs/ten-ways-to-shape-up-your-family-reunion.pdf*

The NDEP also recently developed a discussion guide for a privately-produced docudrama titled "The Debilitator," whose lead character is an African American man who has been diagnosed with type 2 diabetes. Pilot screenings of the film revealed that people wanted to talk after the movie—about their personal experiences and the emotions that accompany living with diabetes and its complications. Therefore, the NDEP developed *New Beginnings: A Discussion Guide for Living Well with Diabetes* to facilitate discussion. For more information, see: *www.ndep.nih.gov/diabetes/pubs/New_Beginnings_2005.pdf*

Finally, DMICC member organizations are also supporting research to translate the results of the DPP to African American communities. For example, researchers are studying various faith-based approaches to deliver the DPP lifestyle intervention.

Discussion of such efforts at DMICC meetings is important to ensure that successful programs are implemented quickly by DMICC member organizations that service this community.

Combating Diabetes in Children: The increasing incidence of diabetes in youth, both type 1 and type 2, has been among the most distressing aspects of the evolving diabetes epidemic. DMICC member organizations are leading the federal effort to understand and fight this disconcerting trend. Because estimates of diabetes incidence and prevalence among U.S. youth are limited, CDC DDT, in collaboration with NIDDK, launched the SEARCH for Diabetes in Youth Study. SEARCH is a multicenter, epidemiological study conducted in geographically dispersed populations that encompass the racial/ethnic diversity of the U.S. The study is designed to characterize the epidemiology of both type 1 and type 2 diabetes, along with the associated complications, levels of care, and impact of diabetes on the daily lives of U.S. children and youth. The first baseline assessment of diabetes rates in children nationwide has been completed, and this allows the study to evaluate trends in diabetes incidence and progression over time. Tracking the burden of diabetes is key to the design and implementation of public health efforts to prevent or control the disease.

One in 14 children in the U.S. between 12 and 19 years of age has pre-diabetes, and many of these children have risk factors for heart disease.[8] In 1999, the DMICC took a decisive step to address this alarming trend and continues to coordinate efforts to protect our children from diabetes and its complications.

Type 1 diabetes is often diagnosed in infancy and childhood. The unrelenting daily burden of managing the disease takes an enormous toll on both the child and the parents. The DMICC plays an important role in coordinating type 1 diabetes research supported by the trans-DHHS *Special Statutory Funding Program for Type 1 Diabetes Research*. This program, established by Congress in 1997 and led by NIDDK, involves many NIH Institutes and Centers, as well as CDC. Type 1 diabetes is a systemic disease addressed by multiple NIH and DHHS entities; the *Special Diabetes Program* has catalyzed and synergized the efforts of this wide range of entities to combat type 1 diabetes and its complications. The *Special Diabetes Program* has been the focus of discussion at several DMICC meetings, and the Committee has coordinated efforts to evaluate the program.

Through support from the *Special Diabetes Program*, numerous large-scale, collaborative research consortia and networks have been established to study type 1 diabetes and its complications. Major research advances have been made possible, including:

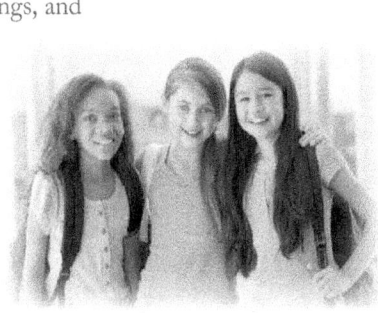

• Development of new continuous glucose monitoring technologies and testing of their use/efficacy in children;

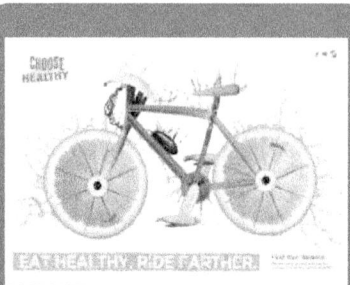

The HEALTHY study, an NIDDK-led clinical trial, is testing whether a middle school-based intervention can prevent risk factors for type 2 diabetes. The intervention consists of changes to school food service and physical education class activities; behavior change activities; and communications and promotional campaigns, such as this poster encouraging kids to get more exercise and eat healthy foods. The HEALTHY study emanated from discussions at a DMICC meeting that focused on ways to combat the increase in type 2 diabetes in children.

- Discovery of multiple genes that affect the risk of type 1 diabetes and that may provide targets for new therapies; and

- Creation of a network to test new therapies to delay the onset or progression of type 1 diabetes.

For more information on the *Special Statutory Funding Program for Type 1 Diabetes Research*, please visit: *www.t1diabetes.nih.gov*

In the battle against type 2 diabetes, the U.S. faces an evolving crisis as more and more youth are diagnosed with the disease, which once was virtually unknown in children. In 1999, the DMICC conducted a meeting focused on type 2 diabetes in children and took decisive steps to address this alarming trend. The input obtained from discussion at this event was critical to the development of NIDDK-supported clinical trials to combat type 2 diabetes in children, such as the following.

- **Treatment Options for Type 2 Diabetes in Adolescents and Youth (TODAY)** is testing different treatment strategies for children ages 10–17 who already have type 2 diabetes.

- The **HEALTHY** study is testing whether a healthy lifestyle intervention targeting middle-schoolers can prevent risk factors for type 2 diabetes. Children are enrolled in the sixth grade and followed for 3 years.

Tackling Diabetes in American Indian Communities: American Indians and Alaska Natives have the highest rates of diabetes in the U.S.[1] In 1997, in parallel with the *Special Statutory Funding Program for Type 1 Diabetes Research*, Congress established the *Special Diabetes Program for Indians* (SDPI), administered by IHS, to address the growing problem of diabetes in those communities. Participation as a DMICC member organization has provided IHS with valuable input on this important program. This involvement also ensured that these communities are included in the design of clinical trials and in efforts to translate research findings to the real world by other DMICC member organizations. In addition, collaboration with NIDDK helped IHS to establish and implement targeted demonstration projects aimed at diabetes prevention and cardiovascular disease risk reduction. Through the SDPI, IHS provided funds to 333 *Community-Directed Diabetes Programs* in 35 states and launched the *Diabetes Prevention Demonstration Project* and the *Healthy Heart Demonstration Project* at 66 sites.

The IHS conducts an ongoing Congressionally-mandated evaluation of the SDPI that describes the evaluation methodology used, programmatic progress made, intermediate outcomes achieved, lessons learned, and best practices emerging from the program. This evaluation has culminated in reports published in 2000, 2004, and

2007. These reports and more information are available online at: *www. ihs.gov/medicalprograms/diabetes*

In September 2008, CDC DDT established 5-year cooperative agreements with 11 tribes and tribal organizations focusing on traditional foods and sustainable ecological approaches in communities. The focus of the 5-year cooperative agreement is to: 1) support community use of traditional foods and sustainable ecological approaches for type 2 diabetes prevention and health promotion in American Indian and Alaska Native communities; and 2) engage communities in identifying and sharing the stories of healthy traditional ways of eating, being active, and communicating health information and support for diabetes prevention and wellness.

To educate the youngest members of this community, CDC DDT and the IHS, in consultation with the Tribal Leaders Diabetes Committee (TLDC), developed an award-winning book series. The books were developed for Native children and encourage a return to traditional ways, including physical activity and healthy eating. The Eagle Books series uses culturally relevant approaches—including the tradition of storytelling—to address the diabetes epidemic in American Indian and Alaska Native communities. Over 2 million books have been distributed in Indian Country, the rest of the U.S., and abroad. In addition, the original watercolors from the books were exhibited at the Smithsonian's National Museum of the American Indian in fall 2008. The CDC DDT also launched the Eagle Books Community Outreach Campaign in fall 2008. From 2008 through 2012, American Indian and Alaska Native communities throughout Indian Country will have an opportunity to host a 4-5 day series of events celebrating the Eagle Books and their culturally-relevant messages about physical activity and healthy eating.

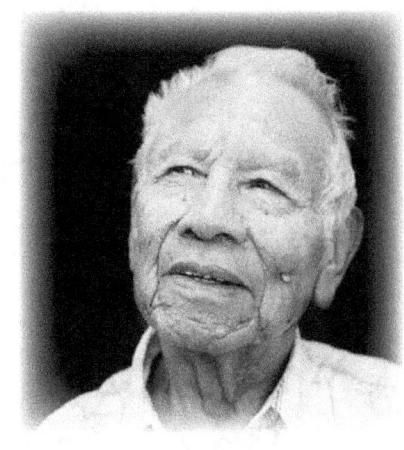

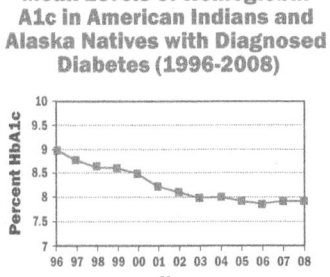

Mean Levels of Hemoglobin A1c in American Indians and Alaska Natives with Diagnosed Diabetes (1996-2008)

Figure 7. Mean levels of HbA1c in American Indians and Alaska Natives with diagnosed diabetes, from 1996–2008.[9] The *Special Diabetes Program for Indians* has helped IHS to improve the health of American Indians and Alaska Natives. Blood glucose control (represented by percent of HbA1c, a test used to measure average blood glucose levels) is improving among people with diabetes in these communities. Each percentage drop translates into a 30 percent reduction in the likelihood of developing complications of diabetes.

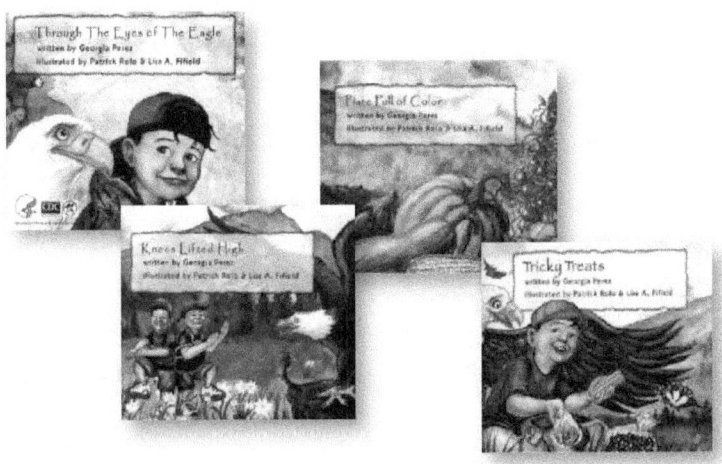

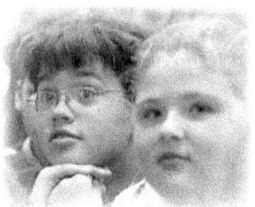

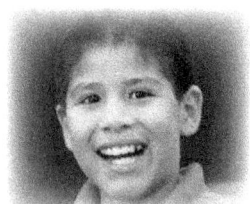

Improving the Delivery of Health Care to Special Populations: DMICC member organizations are leading the way to improve access and delivery of health care to populations at high risk for developing diabetes. For 5 years, CDC DDT and HRSA worked together on the National Diabetes Collaborative, a program designed to improve the treatment of diabetes and pre-diabetes by identifying and defining the best practices in health care. The Collaborative aimed to improve health care delivery systems, increase access to health care, and decrease health disparities among medically underserved populations in federally funded health centers.

The Translating Research Into Action for Diabetes (TRIAD), a CDC DDT-led collaboration including NIDDK and VHA, is a national multicenter study to determine how managed care systems influence the processes and outcomes of diabetes care. TRIAD will assess the level of care provided to people with diabetes, identify the barriers that impede people's access to the care they need, and find new ways to provide better care for diabetes. With this knowledge, TRIAD aims to improve the quality of care and quality of life for people with diabetes and to provide practical information on how to implement effective treatments for people with diabetes in U.S. managed care settings.

Additionally, VHA and DOD have collaborated to overcome obstacles to providing quality health care to patients in remote locations with diabetes. Given the challenges of a growing population with diabetes and the lack of accessible health care, many DMICC member organizations are exploring telemedicine—a way of providing clinical care using telecommunications such as the telephone or Internet. The VHA and DOD validated a system of "tele-retinal" screening using digital images of eyes of patients with diabetes and remote image interpretation. This system has been deployed throughout VHA, especially in rural areas and in primary care clinics.

Ensuring Accuracy and Consistency in Reporting Diabetes Facts

The Importance of Consistent Facts About Diabetes: People are bombarded daily with information about diabetes from the Internet, advertisements, and the media, making it difficult and time-consuming to sort and evaluate the information on which to make important decisions about health. DMICC member organizations, like other health care organizations, have learned from the marketing field: clear and consistent messages are necessary. Messages, including those about diabetes, take many impressions until they "stick," so clear and consistent messages are needed to improve public health. With many diverse federal agency members in attendance, DMICC meetings provide an ideal forum in which to discuss and disseminate consistent messages, facts, and guidelines. This coordination ensures that federal agencies provide the public with the most accurate and helpful information about diabetes prevention and management. Below are a few examples of how DMICC member organizations coordinate and use these consistent facts, guidelines, and messages.

DMICC member organizations coordinate to create and disseminate clear and consistent messages that the public can trust when making decisions about diabetes.

Collaborating To Develop Consistent Facts: The CDC DDT, as the lead federal organization for diabetes surveillance and for tracking trends in diabetes and its complications, develops the *National Diabetes Fact Sheet*—a standard set of diabetes burden estimates that is widely adopted by federal and non-federal entities. The Fact Sheet is the result of collaborations among many DMICC member organizations, including AHRQ, CMS, DHHS OMH, HRSA, IHS, NIDDK, and VHA, as well as professional organizations, information clearinghouses, and patient advocacy groups. The *National Diabetes Fact Sheet* summarizes the latest estimates of Americans with pre-diabetes and with diagnosed and undiagnosed diabetes, as well as other related measures. The information includes data provided by CDC NCHS and is essential for helping those at the federal, state, and local levels understand the health and economic burden of diabetes.

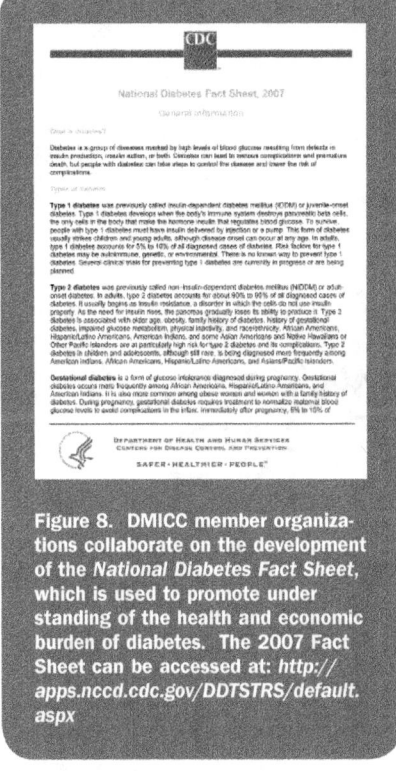

Figure 8. DMICC member organizations collaborate on the development of the *National Diabetes Fact Sheet*, which is used to promote understanding of the health and economic burden of diabetes. The 2007 Fact Sheet can be accessed at: *http://apps.nccd.cdc.gov/DDTSTRS/default.aspx*

Working Together To Standardize Tests: The DCCT demonstrated that improved metabolic control reduces the risk for development of diabetes complications. It established a treatment goal based on the HbA1c test used to measure blood glucose control in the trial. Prior to the DCCT, results from the HbA1c test varied from laboratory to laboratory around the country. To enable health care providers and patients to know if they had achieved the treatment goal that the DCCT had proved so valuable, the tests used to measure HbA1c levels must be reliable and consistent across clinical laboratories. Therefore, CDC DDT

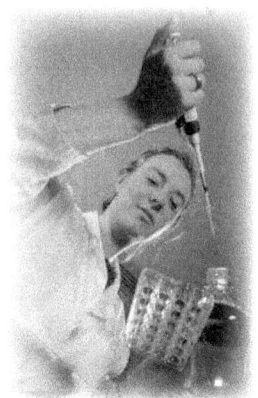

and CDC NCEH, in collaboration with NIDDK and ADA, established the National Glycohemoglobin Standardization Program. This remarkably successful program now certifies over 99 percent of the laboratories measuring HbA1c in the U.S., ensuring standardization and reliability in measures of HbA1c. The standardization of HbA1c measures is essential to public health efforts, such as those of the NDEP, to improve diabetes control, so that clinical laboratory results can be related directly to the results of the DCCT and other studies, and the public can reap the benefits of clinical trials that prove that complications can be delayed or prevented. DMICC member organizations can disseminate information on the importance of long-term blood glucose control, knowing that the public can rely on consistent measures of HbA1c.

Currently, the best predictors of the onset of type 1 diabetes before the appearance of clinical symptoms are the presence of autoantibodies in the blood. The production of autoantibodies reflects abnormal and destructive immune system functioning, which is the underlying cause of type 1 diabetes. The tests that measure these autoantibodies must be reliable and consistent. For example, standardized measurements are crucial to the success of multicenter clinical trials, as different participating laboratories must be able to obtain measurements that are comparable and can be meaningfully analyzed together. The Diabetes Autoantibody Standardization Program, led by CDC NCEH and the Immunology of Diabetes Society in collaboration with NIDDK, is improving the measurement of these autoantibodies and decreasing variation in their measurement among laboratories. Additional efforts by DMICC member organizations are also under way to standardize other important tests used for diabetes research, including measurement of insulin and C-peptide (a byproduct of insulin production).

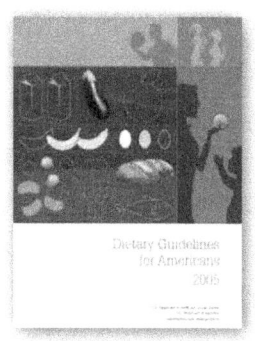

Coordinating To Provide Consistent Messages: The DHHS ODPHP collaborates with USDA and with other DMICC member organizations to provide consistent nutrition messages to the public. The *Dietary Guidelines for Americans*, published every 5 years by DHHS and USDA, provide authoritative advice for people 2 years and older about how good dietary habits can promote health and reduce risk for major chronic diseases such as diabetes. They serve as the basis for federal food and nutrition education programs. DHHS ODPHP also reviews dietary guidance materials to ensure consistency with the Guidelines.

The DHHS also published the *2008 Physical Activity Guidelines for Americans* to provide information and guidance on the types and amounts of physical activity that provide substantial health benefits for Americans aged 6 years and older. The Guidelines were published because being physically active is one of the most important steps that Americans of all ages can take to improve their health. The

Guidelines provide science-based guidance to help Americans improve their health through appropriate physical activity. This effort involved DMICC member organizations.

Generating or Utilizing Consistent Clinical Guidelines: Diabetes clinical guidelines are statements to help the clinician and patient make appropriate decisions about health care; they are tools to improve the processes of care for patients and to provide a consistent quality of care. Guidelines contain recommendations based on evidence from a rigorous systematic review and synthesis of published medical literature. They serve as the basis for accountability, and facilitate learning and the conduct of research. Many DMICC member organizations are actively involved in developing, evaluating, and/or implementing clinical guidelines; coordination is essential to ensure that educational materials and guidelines are consistent and can assist patients and providers in making decisions about diabetes care. Examples of these guidelines follow.

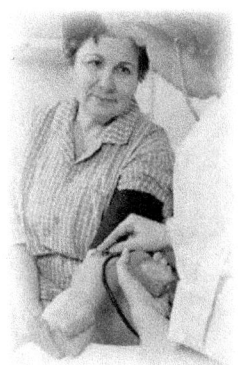

- Through the NDEP, many DMICC member organizations play important roles in disseminating materials based on comprehensive guidelines for many aspects of diabetes prevention and control.

- The NHLBI has led the development of guidelines for management of blood pressure and cholesterol, including in people with diabetes, and the development of clinical guidelines on overweight and obesity. More information is available at: *www.nhlbi.nih.gov/guidelines/index.htm*

- The DOD and VHA collaborated in the development and implementation of evidence-based clinical practice guidelines on diabetes care. These guidelines have been independently determined to be among the most evidence-based in the U.S. (using GRADE) by the American College of Physicians. They are in the public domain (*www.oqp.med.va.gov*).

- The AHRQ's National Guideline Clearinghouse is a public resource that maintains more than 50 evidence-based clinical guidelines related to the management and treatment of diabetes. The AHRQ is working with guideline developers and other stakeholders to improve the guidelines and to convert them into useful measures.

- The NIBIB has participated on a joint committee of the Diabetes Technology Society and the Clinical and Laboratory Standards Institute to develop consensus guidelines for continuous glucose monitoring. These guidelines will be important in the development of new technologies for people with diabetes.

Addressing Opportunities in Diabetes Research

Developing Strategies for Future Diabetes Research: Because the manifestations of diabetes are diverse, the origins of the disease involve many factors, and treatment and prevention are complex and challenging, a wide variety of expertise is required to develop new therapies and prevention measures. Discussions at DMICC meetings provide opportunities for members who are experts in particular aspects of diabetes to share expertise and to learn about different features of the disease. Not only do DMICC discussions strengthen members' knowledge bases, they also promote research collaborations. The discussions are productive and thought-provoking, helping members to identify gaps in the federal diabetes effort and in the knowledge of diabetes. Many current research efforts were topics at DMICC meetings that were further developed and refined by discussions among DMICC members.

The DMICC also plays a key role in coordinating diabetes research strategic planning and evaluation efforts. These efforts are critical to continually assess the diabetes research portfolio and to ensure that the most compelling opportunities for research are addressed. To guide future research efforts in type 1 diabetes, the DMICC, with broad external input, developed *Advances and Emerging Opportunities in Type 1 Diabetes Research: A Strategic Plan*. The Plan, published in August 2006, identifies key research objectives that will guide future NIH efforts to combat type 1 diabetes and its complications.

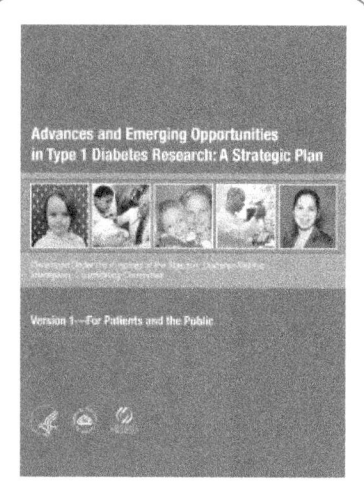

Figure 9. The DMICC developed *Advances and Emerging Opportunities in Type 1 Diabetes Research: A Strategic Plan* to guide type 1 diabetes research (*www.t1diabetes.nih.gov/plan*). The Plan is available in two versions—one for patients and the public and one for the scientific community.

Evaluation of the *Special Statutory Funding Program for Type 1 Diabetes Research*: The DMICC also coordinated a congressionally mandated evaluation of the *Special Statutory Funding Program for Type 1 Diabetes Research*, culminating in a report that describes the collaborative planning process, scientific progress to date, expected future outcomes, and emerging research opportunities that have resulted from research supported by the program. The Evaluation Report is available online at: *www.t1diabetes.nih.gov/evaluation*

Examples of Partnerships Among DMICC Member Organizations To Accelerate Research Progress:

Coordination of Therapeutic Development and Regulation: The NIH plays a key role in research to develop and evaluate new interventions; FDA regulates investigational use of new therapies and assessment of their safety and efficacy prior to market introduction. In efforts to combat diabetes, NIH and FDA are working together on medications, transplantation activities, and efforts to produce an artificial pancreas for patients with type 1 diabetes. These collaborations are through interagency

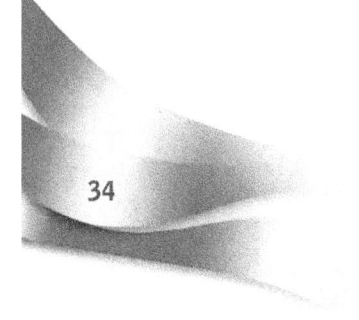

committees, such as the Interagency Artificial Pancreas Working Group; jointly sponsored workshops; and other venues.

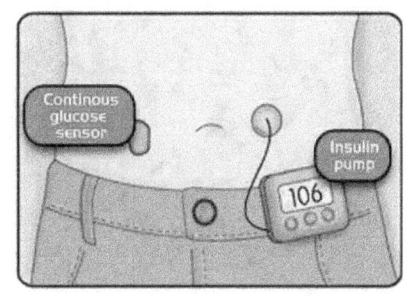

Improving the Translation of Research Into Health Care Improvements: AHRQ's Accelerating Change and Transformation in Organizations and Networks (ACTION) promotes innovation in health care delivery by accelerating the development, implementation, diffusion, and use of research into practice. Several ACTION projects are sponsored by CDC DDT, DOD, and HRSA.

Translating Primary Prevention Into Public Health Programs: DMICC member organizations, including AHRQ and NIH, participated in a CDC DDT meeting of primary prevention experts in 2007, to facilitate interchange between academic experts and federal and state agencies on advancing type 2 diabetes primary prevention on a wider scale. This dialogue among researchers, public health officials, and providers is essential to develop successful public health programs.

Collaborative Research Efforts Among DMICC Member Organizations: Major clinical trials and research programs within the federal diabetes effort are collaborations among several DMICC member organizations. Examples of such efforts follow below.

Diabetes Prevention Program Outcomes Study (DPPOS): The DPPOS is a follow-up study to the DPP clinical trial to examine the long-term effects of diet and exercise and metformin on the delay of type 2 diabetes development. DPP participants are being followed to determine if these interventions are durable and whether prevention or delay of type 2 diabetes translates into a decreased onset of diabetes complications over time. The DPPOS will compare these outcomes for women and men, and by age and ethnicity. The DPPOS is led by NIDDK and includes collaboration with NIA, NEI, NHLBI, NIH Office of Research on Women's Health, NICHD, NCMHD, CDC DDT, and IHS. Additional information about DPPOS can be found in the "Coordinating Federal Efforts to Prevent Type 2 Diabetes" section of this booklet.

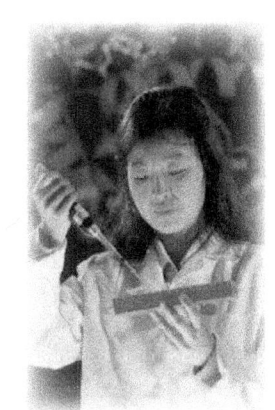

Action to Control Cardiovascular Risk in Diabetes (ACCORD): The ACCORD trial is designed to test three treatment approaches to decrease the high rate of cardiovascular disease among adults with established type 2 diabetes who are at especially high risk for heart attack and stroke. ACCORD is led by NHLBI in collaboration with NIDDK, NIA, and NEI. The CDC DDT funds sub-studies within ACCORD on cost-effectiveness and health-related quality of life. Further information about ACCORD can be found in the "Creation and Support of the National Diabetes Education Program" section of this booklet.

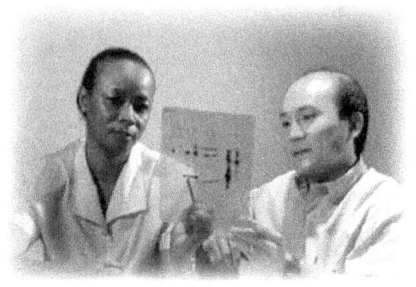

Look AHEAD: Action for Health in Diabetes: Look AHEAD is the largest clinical trial to date to examine the long-term health effects of intentional weight loss in people with type 2 diabetes with respect to cardiovascular events. Look AHEAD was developed in response to a workshop convened by NIH and CDC DDT that concluded that only a randomized clinical trial of intentional weight loss could provide needed guidance on the risks and benefits of weight loss to inform rational clinical and public health policy. Led by NIDDK, this trial is conducted in collaboration with NHLBI, NINR, NIH Office of Research on Women's Health, NCMHD, and CDC DDT.

Type 1 Diabetes TrialNet: Type 1 Diabetes TrialNet is an international consortium of clinical research centers testing novel strategies to prevent type 1 diabetes in people at high risk for the disease, as well as therapies to delay progression of disease in newly-diagnosed patients. To date, TrialNet has developed four prevention studies and eight additional studies to test therapies to halt progression of disease in newly-diagnosed patients. These studies have the potential to have a dramatic impact on our ability to prevent and treat type 1 diabetes. TrialNet is led by NIDDK, in collaboration with NIAID, NICHD, and NCCAM, with support in part from the *Special Statutory Funding Program for Type 1 Diabetes Research*.

The Environmental Determinants of Diabetes in the Young (TEDDY): TEDDY is an international consortium providing a coordinated, multidisciplinary approach to understanding the infectious agents, dietary factors, or other environmental conditions that trigger type 1 diabetes in genetically-susceptible individuals. Identification of these factors will lead to a better understanding of disease and can result in new strategies to prevent, delay, or reverse type 1 diabetes. TEDDY is led by NIDDK, in collaboration with NIAID, NICHD, NIEHS, and CDC DDT, and is supported by the *Special Statutory Funding Program for Type 1 Diabetes Research*.

Clinical Islet Transplantation Consortium (CIT): The CIT has designed eight clinical trials to collaboratively and rigorously study new approaches to islet transplantation in order to improve the safety and long-term success of this therapy in people with type 1 diabetes. Additionally, the Consortium is conducting Phase III trials to support licensure for islets as a cellular therapy. Islet transplantation is a promising therapy that can yield beneficial results for individuals with difficult-to-manage type 1 diabetes, but limitations of the current state-of-the-art must be overcome so more patients can benefit. The CIT is jointly led by NIDDK and NIAID and includes collaboration with CMS. Islet Cell Resource Centers, managed by NCRR and NIDDK, distribute clinical-grade human islets for trials conducted within the CIT. NIDDK and NIAID also support collaborative research consortia testing islet

Through collaboration and partnership among DMICC member organizations, large-scale, critically important research efforts have been undertaken that can have a significant impact on the prevention, treatment, and management of diabetes.

transplantation strategies in non-human primates. These programs are supported by the *Special Statutory Funding Program for Type 1 Diabetes Research*.

The Diabetes Research in Children Network (DirecNet): DirecNet is a multicenter clinical research network conducting studies to understand the factors contributing to—and to develop strategies to prevent—hypoglycemia in children and adolescents with type 1 diabetes. Using new forms of technology, pharmacology, or behavioral interventions, DirecNet is investigating and translating methods of improved glycemic control for children. With support in part from the *Special Statutory Funding Program for Type 1 Diabetes Research*, DirecNet is led by NICHD in collaboration with NIDDK.

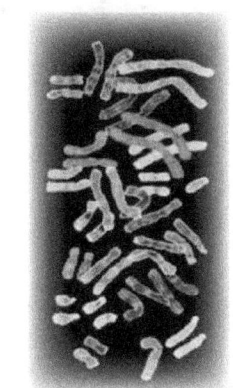

Type 1 Diabetes Genetics Consortium (T1DGC): T1DGC is a large-scale, well-coordinated effort to identify numerous gene combinations that are important in predicting an individual's risk of developing type 1 diabetes or related autoimmune diseases. The success of the T1DGC has led to an increase in the number of genetic elements identified in association with this complex disease. With these exciting new insights, researchers may be able to identify with great precision those individuals at risk for the disease, develop and test prevention-oriented strategies, and design more specific clinical trials to test interventions specifically tailored to patients with similar risk profiles. T1DGC is led by NIDDK in collaboration with NIAID and NHGRI, and is supported by the *Special Statutory Funding Program for Type 1 Diabetes Research*.

Animal Models of Diabetic Complications Consortium (AMDCC): AMDCC is an interdisciplinary consortium designed to develop animal models that closely mimic the human complications of diabetes for the purpose of studying disease pathogenesis, prevention, and treatment. AMDCC has played a critical role in propelling research progress by developing, validating, and distributing animal models with greater fidelity to human type 1 diabetes and its complications to the scientific community. Led by NIDDK in collaboration with NHLBI, AMDCC is supported in part by the *Special Statutory Funding Program for Type 1 Diabetes Research*.

Translating Research Into Action for Diabetes (TRIAD): TRIAD is a 5-year, six-center prospective study of managed care and diabetes quality of care, costs, and outcomes in the U.S. Led by CDC DDT, in collaboration with NIDDK and VHA, TRIAD is an important study because it is the first and largest multicenter study of diabetes quality of care, quality of life, and factors affecting them. The overall goal of the study is to examine the influence of managed care structure on processes and outcomes of diabetes care.

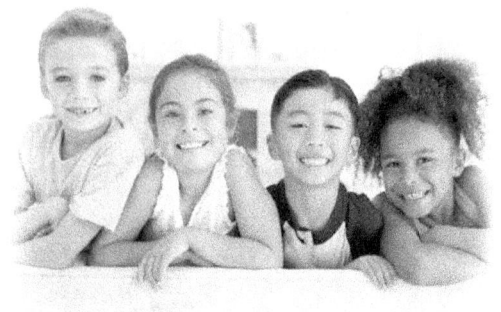

SEARCH for Diabetes in Youth (SEARCH): SEARCH is a multicenter, epidemiological study that examines the current status of diabetes among children and adolescents in the U.S. CDC DDT-led, in collaboration with NIDDK, the study will: 1) develop a uniform classification of types of childhood diabetes (no "gold standard" definitions of types currently exist); 2) estimate the number of new (incidence) and existing (prevalence) childhood diabetes cases by type, age of the child, sex, and racial or ethnic group; 3) describe the clinical characteristics of different types of diabetes in youth and how they evolved; 4) describe the complications of diabetes in children and adolescents; and 5) describe the quality of life of children and adolescents with diabetes. SEARCH is supported in part by the *Special Statutory Funding Program for Type 1 Diabetes Research*.

These programs are critically important research efforts that have the potential to have a significant impact on the prevention, treatment, and management of diabetes and its complications. Some of the efforts, such as ACCORD, have already contributed considerable knowledge about the treatment of type 2 diabetes. Other efforts, such as T1DGC, have resulted in vast new information about the genetic underpinnings of type 1 diabetes—knowledge upon which future research can build to develop novel prevention and treatment strategies. As other research efforts come to fruition, it is expected that they could have an equally important impact on preventing and treating diabetes and its complications. DMICC member organizations have worked together to develop and oversee these large research programs. It has only been through collaboration and partnerships among DMICC member organizations that these research efforts could be undertaken and the potential of basic and clinical diabetes research realized.

LOOKING AHEAD:
FUTURE DMICC ACTIVITIES

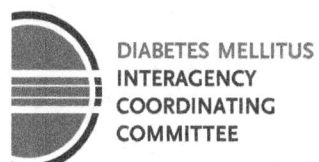

DIABETES MELLITUS
INTERAGENCY
COORDINATING
COMMITTEE

Since its inception, the DMICC has facilitated successful, collaborative diabetes activities among its member organizations. Examples of these efforts include collaborating on activities of the NDEP, coordinating diabetes research supported by the trans-DHHS *Special Statutory Funding Program for Type 1 Diabetes Research*, and coordinating strategic planning efforts in diabetes research. In response to the immense and growing public health burden of diabetes, the DMICC is expanding and strengthening its coordination and collaboration activities. The DMICC is uniquely poised to leverage federal resources, reduce redundancy of effort, and increase public awareness of federal diabetes research, programs, and health information to combat the diabetes epidemic. The DMICC is:

- *Broadening Its Membership:* The DMICC added DOD and USDA to its membership. These new members bring unique expertise and perspective to the activities of the DMICC, as well as new opportunities for collaboration.

- *Focusing Its Members on Strengthening Collaboration:* The DMICC meets to share information and explore potential collaborations. Future meetings will focus on new opportunities for collaboration; establishing new partnerships; and strategic planning to better understand, prevent, and treat diabetes in the U.S.

- *Identifying New Opportunities for Diabetes Research:* Because of the increased public health burden of diabetes in the U.S. and around the world, the DMICC is coordinating a new strategic planning process to identify current advances and future opportunities in diabetes research. This plan is expected to serve as a guide for NIH, CDC, and other DMICC components, as well as for the research community by identifying compelling research opportunities to inform the priority-setting process in the years ahead. Recent DMICC meetings have also led to the identification of new and emerging opportunities for diabetes research.

- *Enhancing Outreach Efforts:* The DMICC is spearheading several new efforts to disseminate information about the Committee and its activities broadly to the public. One of these projects is a new public DMICC Web site that will help disseminate information about the Committee to patients, scientists, policymakers, other federal government entities, and the public; describe major federal diabetes efforts; and link to diabetes health information.

> For more information about the DMICC and its activities, please visit:
> *http://www.diabetescommittee.gov*

These efforts will enable the DMICC to improve the dissemination of information about diabetes, enhance coordination of federal efforts to advance diabetes research, and improve the health of Americans with or at risk for diabetes.

REFERENCES

1. Centers for Disease Control and Prevention. National diabetes fact sheet: general information and national estimates on diabetes in the United States, 2007. Atlanta, GA: U.S. Department of Health and Human Services, Centers for Disease Control and Prevention, 2008.

2. American Diabetes Association. Economic costs of diabetes in the U.S. in 2007. *Diabetes Care* 31: 596-615, 2008.

3. Centers for Disease Control and Prevention, Division of Diabetes Translation, National Diabetes Surveillance System. *http://www.cdc.gov/diabetes*

4. National Institute of Diabetes and Digestive and Kidney Diseases, National Diabetes Information Clearinghouse. *http://diabetes.niddk.nih.gov*

5. Centers for Disease Control and Prevention, National Center for Health Statistics, National Health Interview Survey.

6. Narayan KM, Boyle JP, Geiss LS, Saaddine JB, Thompson TJ. Impact of recent increase in incidence on future diabetes burden: U.S., 2005-2050. *Diabetes Care* 29: 2114-2116, 2006.

7. Narayan KM, Boyle JP, Thompson TJ, Sorensen SW, Williamson DF. Lifetime risk for diabetes mellitus in the United States. *JAMA* 290: 1884-1890, 2003.

8. Williams DE, Cadwell BL, Cheng YJ, Cowie CC, Gregg EW, Geiss LS, Engelgau MM, Narayan KM, Imperatore G. Prevalence of impaired fasting glucose and its relationship with cardiovascular disease risk factors in US adolescents, 1999–2000. *Pediatrics* 116: 1122-1126, 2005.

9. Indian Health Service, National Diabetes Program Statistics, 1996-2008.

ACRONYMS AND ABBREVIATIONS

ACCORD	Action to Control Cardiovascular Risk in Diabetes
ACTION	Accelerating Change and Transformation in Organizations and Networks
ADA	American Diabetes Association
AHRQ	Agency for Healthcare Research and Quality
AMDCC	Animal Models of Diabetic Complications Consortium
CDC	Centers for Disease Control and Prevention
CIT	Clinical Islet Transplantation Consortium
CMS	Centers for Medicare & Medicaid Services
CSR	Center for Scientific Review
CTSA	Clinical and Translational Science Award
DCCT	Diabetes Control and Complications Trial
DDT	Division of Diabetes Translation
DHHS	Department of Health and Human Services
DHHS ODPHP	DHHS Office of Disease Prevention and Health Promotion
DHHS OMH	DHHS Office of Minority Health
DirecNet	Diabetes Research in Children Network
DMICC	Diabetes Mellitus Interagency Coordinating Committee
DOD	Department of Defense
DPP	Diabetes Prevention Program
DPPOS	Diabetes Prevention Program Outcomes Study
FDA	Food and Drug Administration
HRSA	Health Resources and Services Administration
IHS	Indian Health Service
Look AHEAD	Action for Health in Diabetes
mg/dL	milligrams/deciliter
MODY	Maturity-Onset Diabetes of Youth
NCCAM	National Center for Complementary and Alternative Medicine
NCCDPHP	National Center for Chronic Disease Prevention and Health Promotion
NCEH	National Center for Environmental Health
NCHS	National Center for Health Statistics
NCMHD	National Center on Minority Health and Health Disparities
NCRR	National Center for Research Resources
NDEP	National Diabetes Education Program
NEI	National Eye Institute

NHGRI	National Human Genome Research Institute
NHLBI	National Heart, Lung, and Blood Institute
NIA	National Institute on Aging
NIAAA	National Institute on Alcohol Abuse and Alcoholism
NIAID	National Institute of Allergy and Infectious Diseases
NIBIB	National Institute of Biomedical Imaging and Bioengineering
NICHD	*Eunice Kennedy Shriver* National Institute of Child Health and Human Development
NIDA	National Institute on Drug Abuse
NIDCD	National Institute on Deafness and Other Communication Disorders
NIDCR	National Institute of Dental and Craniofacial Research
NIDDK	National Institute of Diabetes and Digestive and Kidney Diseases
NIEHS	National Institute of Environmental Health Sciences
NIGMS	National Institute of General Medical Sciences
NIH	National Institutes of Health
NIMH	National Institute of Mental Health
NINDS	National Institute of Neurological Disorders and Stroke
NINR	National Institute of Nursing Research
NLM	National Library of Medicine
SDPI	Special Diabetes Program for Indians
SEARCH	SEARCH for Diabetes in Youth Study
T1DGC	Type 1 Diabetes Genetics Consortium
TEDDY	The Environmental Determinants of Diabetes in the Young
TLDC	Tribal Leaders Diabetes Committee
TODAY	Treatment Options for Type 2 Diabetes in Adolescents and Youth
TRIAD	Translating Research Into Action for Diabetes
USDA	U.S. Department of Agriculture
VHA	Veterans Health Administration

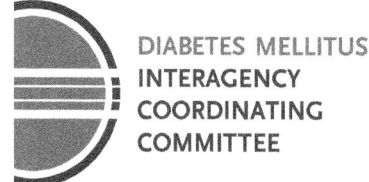

DIABETES MELLITUS
INTERAGENCY
COORDINATING
COMMITTEE

PHOTO CREDITS:

Cover—Photos of children on left bottom: © Chris Schmidt, iStockPhoto

Page 2—© Eddyizm | Dreamstime.com

Page 3—© Cathy Yeulet, 123rf

Page 8—© Graça Victoria, 123rf

Page 21—© Cathy Yeulet, 123rf

Page 22—Top photo: © Don Mace | Dreamstime.com

Page 23—Top photo: © Margarita Borodina, 123rf; Bottom photo: © Monkey Business Images | Dreamstime.com

Page 24—Top photo: © Rohit Seth, 123rf; Bottom photo: © Suprijono Suharjoto | Dreamstime.com

Page 25—© iofoto, 123rf

Page 26—© Cathy Yeulet, 123rf

Page 27—Bottom photo: © Cathy Yeulet, 123rf

Page 29—© Lee Pettet, iStockPhoto

Page 30—Doug Coulson, Ph.D.

Page 32—National Eye Institute, National Institutes of Health

Page 33—© Alexander Raths, 123rf

Page 35—Middle photo: © 2008 Jupiterimages Corporation; Bottom photo: National Eye Institute, National Institutes of Health

Page 36—Richard Nowitz for NIDDK

Page 37—Top photo: Jane Ades, NHGRI; Bottom photo: Richard Nowitz for NIDDK

Page 38—© Cathy Yeulet, 123rf

Page 39—© 2008 Jupiterimages Corporation

ACKNOWLEDGMENT:

Members of the DMICC are thanked for their contributions to this publication.

NIH Publication No. 08-6382
January 2009